Psychological Aspects of Polycystic Ovary Syndrome

John A. Barry

Psychological Aspects of Polycystic Ovary Syndrome

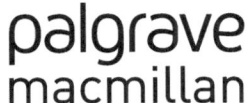

John A. Barry
University College London
London, UK

ISBN 978-3-030-30289-4   ISBN 978-3-030-30290-0   (eBook)
https://doi.org/10.1007/978-3-030-30290-0

This Palgrave Macmillan imprint is published by the registered company Springer Nature Switzerland AG.
The registered company address is: Gewerbestrasse 11, 6330 Cham, Switzerland

I dedicate this book firstly to my late mother, who died shortly before I had finished writing it. No doubt it would have given her great pleasure to know that it had been published and was helping to improve the state of knowledge on PCOS—a subject of significance to my family. Secondly, I dedicate the book to my two sisters, both of whom have PCOS. Without me having ever heard of PCOS at the time, they demonstrated the difficulties of PCOS for me through their teens and early adult life. When later I found out that they shared a health condition characterised by elevated testosterone, I was intrigued. As a recent graduate of psychology, I hadn't learned much about testosterone, except for a little based on 'the mouse model', which as it turns out isn't the best guide to the impact of testosterone on humans. Typical of women with PCOS, my sisters have very rarely even mentioned their condition to me, let alone talked about how it has impacted their lives. I wish more could have been done for them during their early adulthood at a time when they were dating, and perhaps thinking of starting a family. Obviously, I will be extremely glad if my research and this book lead to improvements in this troublesome condition in any way.

I would like to thank Professor Irene Petersen of University College London for her advice on the subtleties of how best to report odds ratios (Chap. 2), and Dr Roger Kingerlee for his comments regarding clinical psychology (Chap. 8).
Last but not least, I would like to thank my wife Louise, whose encouragement has been crucial to the existence of this book.

John A. Barry
Suffolk, England, June 2019

Preface to PCOS Book

September 2011

When I completed my PhD on the psychological aspects of PCOS in 2011, I was very eager to introduce my research to my peers in the field of psychology. I had already done a few presentations to my fellow students and lecturers at City University, London, though often the feedback was 'this is interesting but a bit too medical'. I had a much better reception when presenting to gynaecologists and endocrinologists, because I brought to life some of the experiences they had built up from years of helping women with PCOS, and addressed with research evidence some of the intuitions they had developed about their patients.

So in 2011 I was particularly happy to be presenting the material from my PhD thesis to the European Health Psychology Society (EHPS) in Crete. I was confident that my material was up to standard because my thesis was a 'PhD by publication', that is, it was a compilation of peer-reviewed publications of my research programme, and all of the publications were of respectable quality, and in a couple of cases, very respectable.

This was a big conference spanning five days, and featuring some leading names in health psychology. Although my material was being presented only as a poster rather than as an oral presentation, I was still excited in anticipation of what kinds of reactions I would get, conversations

I would have, collaborations that might be generated. I need not have been so hopeful. Lots of psychologists glanced at my poster and walked on by. Very few showed any more than the merest interest. Much more fascinating to them were the health behaviour models that were being presented and discussed in seminars and workshops. I booked a special feedback session with a leading health psychologist from the US, who told me that my work wasn't really health psychology … maybe more like behavioural medicine. Shouldn't there be more health belief models in my work? I got the point, but couldn't help thinking that her comments reflected an unhealthy obsession in health psychology with trying to make health belief models work better. I couldn't understand why people weren't more interested in testing more tangible bio-psychological models (see Chap. 7). When the conference was over and it came time for me to leave I was disappointed that I had met only one person who was interested in my research, and this person's interest was based solely on the fact that my material was about women's health.

May 2017

Fast forward to the annual British Psychological Society conference in England in May 2017. I had spent most of the intervening years working at the University College London Medical School at the Royal Free Hospital London in Hampstead, first as a research co-ordinator of clinical trials, and then, as a research associate. I put a huge number of hours into PCOS projects that were published, in increasingly in esteemed journals, and was now about to present what I thought was my most exciting project yet—my psychological intervention for women with PCOS.

This was a project I had wanted to do as part of my PhD several years previously, and although it had received ethical approval at City University, the project had stalled in the protracted admin process of approval to recruit participants via the UK's main PCOS charity. Not to worry—some years later, I received ethical approval to recruit at the Royal Free Hospital and University College Hospital. With the help of Brazilian psychotherapist Noelia Leite and other colleagues, our project concluded that androgens can be reduced in PCOS just by using a psychological intervention. This was an exciting discovery.

Now I was standing at the BPS conference. Just as in Crete, I had a poster rather than oral presentation, but never mind. The main thing was that I had a chance to reveal my work to my peers, discuss the implications of the project, and perhaps generate some interest in future research. To my growing dismay almost nobody was interested in my project. The only person who showed interest was a psychologist who said that her female-to-male transsexual clients really liked having PCOS because it gave them a natural boost of androgens. Although of course I found this interesting, I knew that the vast majority of women with PCOS would be perplexed and extremely disappointed to know that not only was there little interest in their condition among psychologists, but that the only psychologist interested thought that PCOS is a good thing.

I'm writing about these experiences to give you some idea of baseline level of interest in PCOS among psychologists in the UK, a level of interest that I believe is replicated globally. There are some exceptions to this rule, notably research teams in the US, Australia, Greece, Italy, and Germany. Despite the excellence of these groups, when you consider the scale of PCOS (at least 1 in 10 women worldwide) and the fact that we are only scratching the surface of the mental health issues related to PCOS (e.g. there are only a handful of studies on interventions for depression in PCOS), then you start to realise that to call PCOS a 'hidden epidemic', as Samuel Thatcher did in 2000, is not far from the truth.

I hope that this book provides a solid platform and guidance for the next generation of PCOS researchers, healthcare workers, and students who will take PCOS research forward. The first three chapters describe and discuss the state of our existing knowledge on different aspects of the mental health and psychobiological aspects of PCOS. The subsequent chapters push the boundaries of what we know about the psychological aspects of testosterone, and provide a theoretical framework as roadmap of the causal relationships between biochemicals and psychology in PCOS. Some of this is speculative, to be sure, but it is the business of science to speculate and generate hypotheses that can then be tested.

Outline of the Chapters in This Book

Chapter 1 is an introduction to some of the key aspects of PCOS. It describes the main medical and psychological features of PCOS and the different types (or phenotypic expressions) of PCOS. It describes the controversy of the competing definitions of PCOS. The possible causes of PCOS are explored, and the chapter also gives a brief introduction to the role of testosterone and insulin in PCOS.

Chapter 2 discusses what is probably the most recognised psychological issue in PCOS—depression. It assesses how well we currently understand the cause of depression in PCOS and the severity. Important methodological issues are discussed and improvements suggested.

Chapter 3 explores anxiety in PCOS, quality of life (QoL), as well as other psychological issues that have been less explored, such as neuroticism. Anxiety has been studied less than depression in PCOS, but in many ways, is just as important as depression in PCOS. Not only is it clinically at least as severe, but the cause of anxiety is possibly more complex than that of depression. Also, the consequences of anxiety are probably more complex too, due to the link between anxiety, adrenal androgens, and PCOS symptoms. Less explored than anxiety is neuroticism, which is a potentially important construct because it appears to provide a conceptual underpinning for psychology and biology in PCOS. Other psychological features of PCOS that have received even less research attention are explored too.

Chapter 4 explores the fascinating role of testosterone and how it impacts women psychologically. The topics include issues that have been widely misunderstood, such as sexual orientation and aggression. No doubt many will be surprised to discover evidence that testosterone is, in fact, a prosocial hormone.

Chapter 5 explores the role of insulin in PCOS and how it is related to testosterone, obesity, and binge eating. Also the fascinating impact of insulin on mood in PCOS will be described.

Chapter 6 outlines ways in which psychology and biology can interact to impact fertility. This chapter also describes evidence related to sexual functioning and satisfaction in women with PCOS, and explores the question of whether there are psychological consequences of oral contraceptive use in PCOS.

Chapter 7 is perhaps the most challenging chapter of the book. In seeking to understand the mechanisms by which psychology is affected by PCOS, four causal pathways are explored. This chapter also explores the fascinating way in which our mental state can impact biology, and the important implications for this in PCOS. Last but by no means least is an exploration of how exposure to testosterone prenatally might be the cause of PCOS.

Chapter 8, the final chapter, brings a spotlight on interventions that might improve mental health in PCOS.

The concluding section takes a look forward at the best next steps in theory and practice for PCOS.

Although the main focus is on psychology, inevitably some medical aspects and treatments are mentioned. For those who are interested in a deeper understanding of the medical aspects, there are excellent textbooks available, and what is written about medical/physiological issues in this book is only the most basic guide, written by a psychologist. No doubt there is exciting new knowledge being created even now, for example, in relation to the role of anti-Müllerian hormone (AMH) and cetrorelix acetate.

Although at the time of writing (June 2019), this book describes a state of knowledge that is very far from complete, it is likely that a more proportionate application of resources to PCOS will deliver correspondingly huge benefits to women who have to live with this difficult condition.

London, UK   John A. Barry

Reference

Thatcher, S. S. (2000). *PCOS (polycystic ovary syndrome): The hidden epidemic.* Perspectives Press.

Contents

List of Figures

1

Introduction to Biological and Psychobiological Aspects of PCOS

Abstract Polycystic ovary syndrome (PCOS) is a complex medical condition in which psychology and biology interact in ways that we are only beginning to appreciate. Understanding the psychological aspects can therefore be a challenging task, and this book aims to map out the full landscape of these issues. To help readers, the first chapter offers a whistle-stop tour of some of the main features of PCOS. Apart from the key medical features (testosterone and insulin), the elephant in the room of PCOS today is the fact that it not only incompletely understood, but experts in this field yet come to a consensus on how it should be defined. Some readers might want to skip ahead to chapters that are focused more purely on psychology, but for the brave, read on.

Keywords Diagnosis of PCOS • Phenotype • Theories of PCOS • Testosterone • Insulin

© The Author(s) 2019
J. A. Barry, *Psychological Aspects of Polycystic Ovary Syndrome*,
https://doi.org/10.1007/978-3-030-30290-0_1

Introduction

Polycystic ovary syndrome (PCOS) is a medical condition that affects 7–20% of women, depending on the diagnostic criteria used (Day et al. 2018). Elevated testosterone levels, or 'hyperandrogenism', is 'perhaps the most consistent and obvious diagnostic feature of PCOS' (Farrell and Antoni 2010, p. 1566), occurring in 60–80% of women with PCOS, depending on the diagnostic criteria. Diagnostic features of PCOS are elevated testosterone (by blood test, or clinical presentation of acne, or hirsutism), menstrual irregularity (nine or fewer periods per year), and multiple cysts on the ovaries.

PCOS is a syndrome, and may be associated with several conditions, though rarely are more than a few present in any one woman with PCOS. Apart from the diagnostic features, other features often seen in PCOS are obesity, insulin resistance (potentially leading to type 2 diabetes), and less commonly male-pattern balding, and dark patches of skin discolouration (acanthosis nigricans). Longer-terms consequences may be endometrial cancer (Barry et al. 2014) and slightly increased cardiovascular risk (Anderson et al. 2014). Most of the problems in PCOS are due to elevated testosterone (hyperandrogenism) and insulin levels (hyperinsulinemia), and it is worth noting that the elevated testosterone is probably due to elevated insulin (Tsilchorozidou et al. 2004).

Research suggests that psychological issues, especially anxiety and depression, are more common in PCOS than in healthy women (Barry et al. 2011). The exact cause of these issues is complex, but is likely to be at least in part due to the distressing symptoms of PCOS.

The estimated annual healthcare cost of PCOS in the UK is at least £237 million (Ding et al. 2018), with most of these costs being associated with direct and indirect aspects of diabetic care. A similar costing has not been conducted for the US recently, but Azziz (2005) estimated the annual cost at $4.36 billion, with 40% of that cost being associated with diabetes. Because obesity is a key factor in the development of diabetes, especially in PCOS (Sam 2007), reduction of obesity should be a key target for anyone interested in PCOS.

There can be little doubt that it is distressing to have a condition like PCOS. Typical symptoms are fertility problems, excess hair growth (hirsutism), acne, and weight gain (Escobar-Morreale 2018). Given that testosterone—often called the 'male sex hormone'—is one of the key features of PCOS, and that testosterone has a masculinising effect on women (and men), it is little wonder that the title of an early paper on PCOS was 'The Thief of Womanhood' (Kitzinger and Willmott 2002). As well as the impact on femininity, a woman diagnosed with PCOS also needs to take on board the longer-term risks of type 2 diabetes, endometrial cancer, and cardiovascular disease. Patients sometimes complain that there is a lack of professional help, support, and research, which can lead to a sense that they are, according to one small study, 'walking around blindfolded' (Busby and Simpson 2019). It's no wonder that some women worry excessively after being diagnosed with PCOS (Azziz 2014), but as we will see in this book not everything about PCOS is inevitably gloomy.

The remainder of this chapter will outline what PCOS is, and what we know of the causes. In one way this is a logical place to start a book on PCOS, but there are two caveats here. Firstly, those interested in the psychological aspects of PCOS will find this first chapter, being focused on technical and physiological aspects of PCOS, less relevant. On the other hand, anyone interested in understanding the psychological aspects of PCOS—for themselves or for patients—should be aware of some of the basic issues. Secondly, any readers can be forgiven for finding the lack of consensus regarding diagnosis, and the lack of certainty regarding the cause of PCOS, somewhat unrewarding to read about. All readers might take comfort in the recent evidence that, despite the lack of consensus and certainty, we can be pretty sure that there is a genetic reality to PCOS, as shown by the shared underlying genetic basis that is not rigidly bound by diagnostic criteria and phenotype (Day et al. 2018).

Phenotypes of PCOS: Definitions and Controversies About Diagnoses

Although polycystic ovaries were first described by Italian scientist Vallisneri in 1721 (Szydlarska et al. 2017), it was largely forgotten until the 1930s, and then renamed after its rediscoverers as Stein-Leventhal syndrome. Even then, it still wasn't until the invention of the ultrasound scanner in the 1980s and consensus of diagnosis in the early 1990s that PCOS was recognised on a wider scale in women of reproductive age.

When attempting to diagnose with precision something that is complex, it is important that we first clearly define what it is we are trying to diagnose. PCOS is today seen as a heterogeneous syndrome where a range of symptoms may be present or absent, and may overlap with other conditions. In their influential paper, Hunter and Sterrett state that PCOS 'is perhaps best viewed as a spectrum of symptoms, pathologic findings and laboratory abnormalities' (Hunter and Sterrett 2000, paragraph 10). PCOS can be difficult to conceptualise, even for experts, as shown by the fact that there have been several different ways of diagnosing it over the years. The issue remains somewhat confusing—not least because you don't need to have polycystic ovaries to have a diagnosis of PCOS—but I will try to make it as simple as possible below.

Identifying types, or more specifically *phenotypes* (observable physiological characteristics created by the genes and environment), is a complex task because there appears to be a range of expression of PCOS. Diamanti-Kandarakis et al. (2006) note that one of the problems of research in this area is that there is not simply one type of PCOS, and genes for one type (e.g. obese/anovulatory) may not contribute to the development of another (e.g. lean/ovulatory). In other words, the fact that there are several overlapping phenotypes makes it difficult to identify the underlying genotype(s).

The first widely accepted diagnostic criteria for PCOS was by the Zawadski and Dunaif (1992). This required two criteria for diagnosis: oligoovulation (eight or fewer periods per year) and androgen excess (clinical or biochemical). Subsequently an expanded set of criteria emerged, which included the presence of polycystic ovaries (multiple small cysts on the ovaries, seen using an ultrasound scan) as one of the criteria. Although its inclusion no doubt adds face validity, polycystic ovaries are not a necessary condition for a PCOS diagnosis with either the National Institutes of Health (NIH) or the more recent Rotterdam diagnostic criteria (2003), or the (less commonly used) Androgen Excess Society criteria (Azziz et al. 2006). The Rotterdam criteria were created by the European Society for Human Reproduction and Embryology and the American Society for Reproductive Medicine (Rotterdam ESHRE/ASR 2003) and are the most widely used in the UK. But not everyone accepts the Rotterdam criteria, for example, Azziz (2006). The Rotterdam criteria are more inclusive and suggest a greater prevalence of PCOS (up to 12% of women) than the NIH definition (up to 8%) (Norman et al. 2007). Note that all diagnoses stipulate the exclusion of related disorders, such as congenital adrenal hyperplasia (CAH) or virilising tumours (tumours which secrete androgen).

Taking the main diagnostic features of PCOS (oligo anovulation, elevated testosterone/hirsutism, and polycystic ovaries), there are 16 different types of PCOS (phenotypes) that can be potentially identified; six ways of diagnosing PCOS by the NIH criteria; and ten ways by the Rotterdam criteria (Azziz et al. 2009). Some experts (Dunaif and Fauser 2013) argue that there are really two main phenotypes: those with polycystic ovaries and subfertility, and those with more metabolic risk (related to insulin resistance). Others note that there is also a less common *lean* type of PCOS, characterised by low body fat and elevated testosterone, thus in general we might say that there are three main phenotypes of PCOS.

Diagnosing PCOS is not just an academic exercise, but has implications for the treatment of PCOS. The problem caused by a lack of clarity (or consensus) over diagnosis is demonstrated when we are trying to assess the impact of PCOS longitudinally, as shown by studies of cancer in PCOS. Because cancer is a disease that typically has a long course, we usually see it only in later life. So if we study cancer in PCOS today, we are assessing women in their 50s or older, who may have been through a healthcare system at a time when PCOS was not widely recognised; thus, their PCOS was missed, or was diagnosed using criteria that are not recognised today (Barry et al. 2014). This means in much of the existing research on the relationship between PCOS and cancer, relying on the accuracy of PCOS diagnosis from decades ago, we usually cannot be sure that the control group definitely don't have PCOS, and we cannot be sure that the women in the PCOS would get a diagnosis using current criteria. This is true even of very good studies today using registers containing many thousands of women (e.g. Cesta et al. 2016). The average age of diagnosis of endometrial and ovarian cancer is the early 60s, which means that a woman who was diagnosed with PCOS 30 years ago while aged 25 might today be too young to have a diagnosis of endometrial and ovarian cancer. However, in another decade or two we will begin to have much better data on which to assess cancer risk in PCOS.

There are important distinctions to be made in the types of problem experienced by women with PCOS, for example, insulin-resistant versus non-insulin-resistant (Acien et al. 1999) but there is no consensus as to whether these basic dichotomies constitute types.

It is interesting that insulin resistance does not figure in the NIH and Rotterdam definitions despite the high rates of insulin resistance seen in PCOS and the fact that insulin leads to increased testosterone levels in PCOS (Buffington et al. 1991). On the other hand, such an inclusion might overlap and there could be dual diagnosis with insulin-related conditions, especially syndrome X.

The most immediately obvious distinction that has some agreement amongst clinicians is the distinction between the obese type that features insulin resistance (and possibly hyperandrogenism) and the lean type that is often hyperandrogenic. The lean type is far less common; in Spain the estimated rate of PCOS in lean women is 5.5% (Barclay and Murata 2006). A review of the features of lean women with PCOS by Goyal and Dawood (2017) found that the lean phenotype is less likely as compared to other women with PCOS to be diabetic, and have insulin-resistant or metabolic abnormalities. Leans have less visceral fat than other women with PCOS, and are less likely to be anovulatory than obese women with PCOS.

Although there is broad agreement that there are two or three main types of PCOS, there remains speculation about the degree to which there are other distinct categories of PCOS, for example, types based on three differential responses to human corticotropin-releasing hormone suggested by Kondoh et al. (1999). Differences in type can also be seen cross-culturally. For example, women from the Pacific Islands with PCOS are less inclined to acne and hirsutism than European women (Williamson et al. 2001). There is also the question of and the degree to which there is comorbidity between PCOS and metabolic syndrome ('syndrome X'), and how to categorise cases where the overlapping of syndromes occurs.

Diamanti-Kandarakis et al. (2008) describe two types of PCOS which they suggest are manifest from birth. The possibility of diagnosis at birth represents a significant advance, not least because early diagnosis offers the important possibility of early treatment. The first phenotype is expressed in low birth weight, but the weight is regained within 12 months. This pattern of development is called 'postnatal catch-up growth'. Premature adrenarche (activity of adrenals at puberty) occurs, and at adolescence hyperandrogenism and anovulation occur, but with normal ovarian morphology. The second type is overweight at birth, is obese in childhood, and experiences the complete 'triad' of problems of PCOS, that is, hyperandrogenism, anovulation, and polycystic ovaries (see also section on PCOS in childhood, below).

More longitudinal research in this area is necessary, and a good example of the insights that can be gained by taking a longitudinal approach is a study by Franceschi et al. (2009). They followed up 46 adolescent girls who had precocious (early) puberty with no identifiable pathological cause, and found that at age 18 (±3 years) 32% of them had PCOS, mainly characterised by polycystic ovaries and elevated testosterone (either by clinical signs, e.g. hirsutism, or assay). Future follow-ups of this cohort will give us further useful information, but the evidence so far suggests that diagnosis of a specific type of PCOS (polycystic ovaries + hyperandrogenism) might be possible at a young age. The importance of this is that the earlier the phenotype is identified, the earlier available treatment approaches can be initiated. In the case of this particular phenotype, it would seem likely that anti-androgens (e.g. spironolactone) would be more appropriate than insulin sensitisers (e.g. metformin). However, without the knowledge of the type of PCOS that is likely to develop from precocious puberty, there would be no way of deciding whether treatment with either anti-androgens or insulin sensitisers would be more appropriate.

One problem facing the creation of a typology of PCOS is that many cases need to be seen in a single study before different categories become obvious, but research in PCOS has been hampered by small sample sizes (Escobar-Morreale et al. 2005). Although perhaps 10% of women have PCOS, because a smaller proportion have each type (e.g. only perhaps 5.5% of women have lean-type PCOS), the sample sizes required for an epidemiological study are quite large. Most of the research done in Europe (including my own research) used the Rotterdam criteria to diagnose PCOS in all cases, and much of the research done in the US uses the

NIH definition. The limitations of these (and other) definitions should be borne in mind, as well as the difficulty of comparing research that uses different definitions.

As can be seen, the diagnosis of PCOS and the PCOS phenotypes is a work in progress. The most likely reason that there are different PCOS phenotypes is because of the complexity of interactions between nature and nurture, including gene expression (see *epigenetics* below). This is an aspect of PCOS that needs more research.

The Relevance of Cysts in PCOS

The inclusion of polycystic ovaries in the Rotterdam definition not only makes sense at face value, but also makes sense biochemically because the cysts (immature ovarian follicles) prevent the conversion of testosterone to estradiol (or E2, the main estrogen), thus disrupting an important step in the fertility process. In the PCOS ovary an abnormal number of ovarian follicles develop, but don't develop to maturity. Mature follicles contain granulosa cells that express aromatase, but in polycystic ovaries this stage of development is not reached (Gougeon 1996).

Possible Causes of PCOS: Evolution, Genetics, Environmental Endocrine Disruptors, Prenatal Development

Although our understanding of PCOS has grown over the past few decades, the cause remains unclear. Like diabetes, the cause is likely to involve both genetics and the environment.

Theoretical Perspectives: The Evolutionary Perspective

The first documented description of polycystic ovaries was made by Vallisieri in 1721 (cited in Eggers et al. 2007) in relation to infertility, and until very recently PCOS was seen as solely a fertility problem (Hunter and Sterrett 2000). Fertility problems have existed for as long as mankind has existed, and the social importance of infertility is evidenced by the prevalence of fertility rituals and fertility goddesses from mankind's earliest history and across cultures (Gelis 1989; Schenker 2000). Given that infertility is by its nature a condition that acts against being inherited, its historical prevalence suggests that its cause is not primarily genetic, and may therefore have environmental causes.

Some authors have speculated that—paradoxically—there is adaptive value in being infertile, whether due to PCOS or other reasons. These evolutionary explanations are included here because they have value on an academic level, but note that some people may take offence to them on a personal level. Eggers et al. (2007) draw upon the kin selection hypothesis to explain how having PCOS offers a selective advantage. The kin selection hypothesis (Hamilton, 1963, 1964a, b) suggests that a person might help the offspring of a relative to survive, and because the helper shares genes with the relative's offspring, at least some part of the helper's genes survive into the next generation. Because raising human newborns is more demanding in time and energy than raising newborns in other species, it is especially useful for the survival of the human child to have a 'helper at the nest'. Amongst primates, this helper is most likely to be nulliparous females, regardless of age (Hrdy 1999). In humans, these females may be women who have not been reproductively successful in their own right, but they may show interest in caring for the child of a sister, cousin, or niece. Indeed, this provides an explanation for the adaptive value of old age in women too; 'the grandmother hypothesis' suggests that postmenopausal women have an important adaptive role (Hawkes et al. 1998). With help from non-reproductive female relatives, fertile women are more free to reproduce more frequently thus increasing the representation of the family's genes—including the helper's—in the gene pool. Having links to more children also benefits the helpers in increasing their chances of having someone to take care of them when they are ill or old.

The metabolic abnormality often seen in PCOS that leads to weight gain can also confer an adaptive advantage, according to Shaw and Elton (2008). They suggest that the tendency to store fat confers a survival advantage on women during times when food is scarce. This advantage also applies to the fetus when such women are pregnant, consistent with the greater birth weight sometimes seen in newborns born to mothers with PCOS.

There is also evidence for a male phenotype for PCOS. This isn't as counterintuitive as it might at first sound. After all, PCOS runs in families, and is related to testosterone and diabetes, both of which are common to men. A meta-analysis found that brothers of women with PCOS are at increased risk of hypertension ($p < 0.00001$) and higher systolic BP than controls ($p = 0.02$) (Yilmaz et al. 2018). However, this was based on a small number of studies, and further research is needed.

A more positive interpretation of the adaptive value of PCOS is made by Gersh and Perella (2018), who suggest that in ancient times, women having slightly higher testosterone and slightly lower fertility were probably stronger, bolder and braver than the average woman.

The Genetic Perspective

Most experts agree that PCOS is to some degree inherited, though the precise mechanism isn't clear yet. Identifying candidate genes has not always been successful, and the interaction of nature and nurture is particularly complex in PCOS. At present there is some encouraging news about the relevance of the *DENND1A* gene in PCOS, which is associated with the regulation of ovarian androgen biosynthesis (Dapas et al. 2019).

In the general population of healthy women, 40% of the variance in testosterone levels is inherited (Harris et al. 1998), and more so in white people than black (Hong et al. 2001). The rate of inheritance is likely to be at least this high for PCOS, and Legro et al. (1998) have found that 50% of sisters of women with PCOS have elevated free or total testosterone. In their study of PCOS in twins, Jahanfar et al. (2004) found that polycystic ovaries are less heritable than androgen and insulin levels. In a PCOS twin study (1332 monozygotic and 1873 dizygotic twins), Vink et al. (2006) found a concordance rate for PCOS symptoms of 0.71 for monozygotic (identical) twins compared to 0.38 for dizygotic (nonidentical) twins and other sisters, indicating a contribution of heredity in PCOS. Dunaif and Thomas (2001) found that 50% of sisters of women with PCOS have polycystic ovaries and hyperandrogenemia. Kahsar-Miller et al. (2001) found that 24–32% of first-degree relatives (mothers, sisters, daughters) of women with PCOS also have PCOS. The prevalence rate of PCOS also varies by ethnicity; Williamson et al. (2001) found that PCOS is more prevalent in Indian women and less prevalent in Chinese women than European women. However, the specific genetic factors associated with PCOS are complex and as yet poorly understood.

Diamanti-Kandarakis et al. (2006) suggest that there have been five obstacles to understanding the contribution of genetics to PCOS. Firstly, there is the problem of overlapping phenotypes (outlined above). Secondly, there is the difficulty of finding evidence of heredity in a condition that works against having children. Thirdly, evidence for the phenotype can only be seen in women of reproductive age. Fourthly, it is generally thought possible only to observe the phenotype in females, not in males. Finally, inherited conditions can usually be modelled in mice—a very useful process known as 'genetic mapping'. However, PCOS is not known to occur spontaneously in any species other than humans, thus precluding the use of genetic mapping. So for many years researchers had tried but failed to make progress in identifying a gene that significantly contributes to the development of any one specific type of PCOS. Despite these obstacles, a recent study of 10,074 women with PCOS and 103,164 control women has found 13 loci which demonstrate a common structure between not only NIH- and Rotterdam-diagnosed PCOS, but self-reported PCOS (Day et al. 2018). The analysis revealed loci related to depression, hyperandrogenism, gonadotropin regulation, obesity, fasting insulin, type 2 diabetes, lipid levels, coronary artery disease, menopause timing, male-pattern balding, and also the male phenotype of PCOS. This means that although the phenotype remains complex, we can at least be somewhat assured that there is a verifiable genotypic basis to PCOS.

This complexity of the possible causes of PCOS is demonstrated by studies of epigenetics. For example, Lambertini et al. (2017) compared the global methylation patterns in umbilical cord blood of newborns delivered to PCOS women and healthy women. Their findings suggest a 'PCOS epigenomic superpathway' triggered by the upregulation of the estrogen receptor gene in utero. Epigenetics is a fascinating topic, offering a fresh perspective on the dynamic interaction of nature and nurture, and more epigenetic research is needed in relation to PCOS.

The Environmental Perspective

PCOS is not simply an inherited condition; it appears to follow the diathesis-stress model, that is, it is a genetic syndrome most likely to become manifest under certain environmental conditions. One of the principal stressors is diet. In their review of the genetic and molecular basis of PCOS, Escobar-Morreale et al. (2005) conclude that the phenotype is modified by ethnicity, diet, and lifestyle factors. The modern Western diet (plentiful, and high in calories, saturated fats, sugars, and carbohydrates) is well established as a risk factor for PCOS. A lack of exercise compounds the problem caused by diet. Unsurprisingly then, interventions that improve diet and exercise tend to have good outcomes for women with PCOS although long-term outcomes need more research (Moran et al. 2006). (See Chap. 8 of this book). A meta-analysis by Miazgowski et al. (2019) found that although prevalence rates of PCOS have been stable across EU since 1990, the prevalence of PCOS is much lower in Western Europe than Central or Eastern Europe. The most likely reason for this difference is the better health behaviours and healthcare in Western Europe. This demonstrates the importance of these environmental factors to PCOS.

Other environmental factors that have been suggested to trigger PCOS are medication, viruses, stress, and endocrine disruptors.

Valproic acid is a medication used to treat epilepsy, bipolar disorder, and migraine headaches. There is some debate over whether long-term use of valproic acid can cause PCOS, and that discontinuation will reduce PCOS symptoms (Isojarvi et al. 1998). However, this hypothesis has been contested on the grounds that the evidence is retrospective and relies on small samples (Genton et al. 2001). (See also the section on bipolar disorder in Chap. 3 of this book.)

There is evidence that adenovirus-36 (Ad-36) causes obesity in rhesus and marmoset monkeys (Dhurandhar 2002) and is related to obesity in humans (Dhurandhar 1997). Although there is no evidence that Ad-36 is associated with the development of PCOS, its potential as a contributor deserves research.

Eggers and Kirchengast (2001) suggest that psychological stress may contribute to the development of PCOS. This is possible via a number of psychological and behavioural pathways; for example, if an adolescent girl engages in comfort eating due to stress, this may cause obesity (Keski-Rahkonen et al. 2007), and obesity at puberty is a known risk for PCOS. Stress is a sufficient cause for the development of functional hypothalamic secondary amenorrhea (FHSA), a condition characterised by elevated adrenal androgens (Gallinelli et al. 2000). Similarly, psychological distress may activate the adrenal glands releasing dehydroepiandrosterone sulphate (DHEAS), which will raise testosterone levels, especially in PCOS patients whose adrenal glands are hyperresponsive to the stress hormone Adrenocorticotropic hormone (ACTH) (Moran et al. 2004). However, although stress is potentially a risk factor for PCOS, the contribution of adrenal androgens alone is unlikely to be sufficient to cause the range and severity of metabolic and endocrinological problems that constitute any PCOS phenotype.

Endocrine disruptors are chemicals found in the environment that can alter the endocrine system of humans and other animals. There are many such chemicals, and perhaps the one that has caused the most concern is bisphenol A (BPA). BPA is a chemical widely used in manufacturing, and despite being discovered in 1936 to be estrogenic (i.e. mimics the action of estrogen), it is still used to line tin cans and plastic containers. BPA can 'leach' from such containers due to high heat or general wear and tear, and can be found in the urine of 93% of Americans. BPA becomes inactive in the human body within a few hours, though some people may be more vulnerable due to, for example, a slow metabolism. Kandaraki et al. (2011) found an association between serum BPA levels and increased testosterone, androstenedione, and insulin resistance in 71 women with PCOS. Lazurova et al. (2018) found higher levels of BPA in the urine of 86 women with PCOS compared to 32 healthy controls. However, not all research supports the PCOS/BPA link (e.g. Li et al. 2011) and a statement by the Endocrine Society (Gore et al. 2015) concluded that the evidence for an impact of endocrine disruptors on PCOS was limited by small sample sizes and reliance on evidence from animal studies which don't necessarily generalise to humans. Nonetheless, the problem of endocrine disruptors is potentially large enough that the European parliament in April 2019 approved a resolution to take action to protect human health and the environment from this problem.

The Fetal Environment

A special case of possible environmental causes of PCOS is the fetal environment. Barker (2004) proposed that some diseases of adulthood may have their origin in conditions in the fetal environment, and women with PCOS have been found to have much higher levels of testosterone than controls during the first trimester (Hu et al. 2007). Although placental aromatase is traditionally thought to protect the fetus from raised maternal testosterone (Abbott et al. 2002), the results of animal research suggest otherwise. For example, Resko and Ellinwood (1984), Resko et al. (1987) gave doses of testosterone (10 to 15 mg) to pregnant rhesus monkeys. The doses were high for a female fetus but normal for a male, and the resulting female offspring were twice as likely to develop PCOS than a control group of untreated females. Based on this and similar evidence, Dumesic et al. (2007) hypothesise that PCOS develops as a result of exposure to abnormally high levels of testosterone prenatally.

Insulin resistance in PCOS offers another possible pathway for prenatal androgenisation, because aromatase activity is inhibited by insulin (Nestler 1990). Aromatase normally converts testosterone into estradiol, and interference with this process could create an androgen-rich fetal environment. However, it remains unclear how much maternal testosterone contributes to fetal levels in human pregnancies, or whether it is possible to control maternal testosterone levels. Vanky et al. (2004) found that taking metformin—an insulin sensitiser—reduced pregnancy complications (e.g. premature birth) in women with PCOS without reducing testosterone levels. Similarly, Glueck et al. (2004) did not find that metformin significantly reduced testosterone during PCOS pregnancies, though they found that testosterone levels remained fairly stable over the three trimesters (56.5, 54.3, and 63.8 ng/dl) on metformin.

A review by Filippou and Homburg (2017) suggests that PCOS is caused by elevated prenatal androgen exposure. There is controversy over the mechanism by which prenatal androgen exposure occurs. It might be genetic, possibly triggering the prenatal ovaries to produce androgen (Franks et al. 2006). Or the pathway might be biological—a transfer of testosterone from the mother's circulation to the fetus (Barry et al. 2010). However, the evidence for the former is weak, and the evidence for the latter is necessarily indirect, given the obvious limitations of experimental work in humans. One the other hand, the mounting evidence (e.g. Barrett et al. 2018) suggests that PCOS is caused by exposure to elevated testosterone prenatally, whatever the mechanism for this turns out to be. The possible mechanisms and pathways are explored in Chap. 7 of this book.

AMH and Prenatal Androgenisation

There are probably several ways in which prenatal androgenisation of the fetus might occur. A recent explanation is that anti-Müllerian hormone (AMH) is implicated in the prenatal origins of PCOS (Tata et al. 2018). Tata et al. found higher maternal serum concentration of AMH in pregnant women with PCOS compared to healthy controls. They explored this phenomenon further using an animal model; when pregnant mice were injected with AMH, it caused increased maternal testosterone, reduced conversion of testosterone to estradiol in the placenta, and resulted in a PCOS phenotype in adult mice offspring.

How does this mechanism work? Well, AMH helps the process of converting the undifferentiated / female fetus to male. Previous research has found AMH in the follicles of the human ovary, the same follicles that are the 'cysts' in PCOS (Pellatt et al. 2010). AMH contributes to the development of the follicles, and helps in the selection of the dominant follicle by competing with the action of aromatase and follicle stimulating hormone (FSH). The increased number of immature follicles in the PCOS ovary produce high levels of AMH, and the high levels of AMH have been implicated in causing menstrual irregularity in PCOS (Homburg and Crawford 2014). During pregnancy, excess AMH causes prenatal androgenisation of the fetus. This is partly due to AMH causing the elevation of maternal testosterone levels, and also—although AMH does not cross the placental barrier—Tata et al. (2018) found that it inhibits the expression of substances in the placenta that convert androgens to estrogens, which in effect increases the availability of testosterone to have organisational effects on the fetus. These findings have caused much excitement, especially because Tata et al. found that they could reduce the PCOS phenotype in their mice by administration of a gonadotropin-releasing hormone (GnRH) antagonist, cetrorelix acetate (or *Cetrotide*). Clinical trials of cetrorelix in women with PCOS are sure to follow, though given the time and resources needed for work of this kind, talk of an imminent cure for PCOS would be premature, especially as any prenatal (organisational) effects would be permanent (see Chap. 7).

Evidence of PCOS in Childhood

If PCOS has its origins in prenatal development, then it stands to reason that there could be signs of PCOS evident in childhood. Diamanti-Kandarakis et al. (2008) review the literature on the early expression of PCOS. They suggest that signs can be seen at birth (high birth weight or low birth weight, with postnatal catch-up within a year) and the classic symptoms of PCOS begin to show in adolescence. Diamanti-Kandarakis et al.'s description of postnatal weight catch-up as an early sign of PCOS is almost entirely based on animal studies, for example, sheep experiencing supraphysiological doses of testosterone (Manikkam et al. 2004), and is thus not necessarily applicable to humans with only moderately elevated testosterone, though there is research evidence in humans that postnatal catch-up in early childhood is associated with many problems at three years of age, including obesity and insulin resistance (Iniguez et al. 2006).

Precocious (early onset) puberty is also seen as a sign of the potential development of PCOS (e.g. Franceschi et al. 2009). However, diagnosing PCOS at puberty can lead to false-positive results because some of the signs of a normal puberty are similar to those of PCOS (acne, irregular menstrual cycles) (Diamanti-Kandarakis et al. 2008), and in puberty it is not unusual to see multiple cysts on at least one ovary in 10% of normally menstruating adolescents. Also, because of the increase in growth hormone in adolescence, insulin resistance is not uncommon. For these reasons the presence of four of five criteria (menstrual irregularity, acne or hirsutism, elevated testosterone, insulin resistance, polycystic ovaries) is recommended to diagnose PCOS in adolescence (Sultan and Paris 2008).

Franks (2008) suggests that the rise in childhood obesity is responsible for triggering symptoms of PCOS, and of exacerbating insulin-related problems at adolescence. Franks also suggests that elevated serum androgens should be considered the hallmark of PCOS in adolescents. However, Diamanti-Kandarakis et al. (2008) caution against biochemical measures of testosterone in diagnosis because of the perceived low reliability of some types of testosterone assays.

The Impact of Testosterone

Masculinising Effects in PCOS and CAH

Broadly speaking, the effects of elevated testosterone are known as *hyperandrogenism.* Elevated testosterone is one of the characteristics of PCOS, and there is growing evidence that PCOS is associated with various physical and psychological conditions, largely thought to be caused by elevated testosterone. It should be noted, however, that it is normal and healthy for women to have some testosterone in their bodies. Indeed, androgen receptor cells in the ovary are critical to healthy ovulation (Astapova et al. 2019). As with many things in life, balance is the key, and a healthy balance between estrogen and testosterone in women (around 10:1) can be visualised as a relationship similar to the 'yin-yang' of Taoism (Barry and Owens 2019). Elevated testosterone has been found to have various physical and psychological effects in a condition with some similarities to PCOS, classical congenital adrenal hyperplasia (CAH). CAH is a relatively rare condition (1 in 15,000 live births) caused by enzymatic deficiency in the glucocorticoid pathway and resulting in overproduction of adrenal androgens prenatally (Miller and Levine 1987) and continuing until identified and treated, usually shortly after birth in females. The levels of androgens experienced by the fetus with CAH are difficult to estimate but probably much higher than seen in the fetus in a PCOS pregnancy. Forest et al. (1981) found that testosterone in the fetal environment of girls with CAH was in same range as that of normal male pregnancies at their highest point during the 'testosterone surge' of prenatal weeks 8–24 (Smail et al. 1981). In CAH these levels are high enough to cause females to be born with ambiguous genitalia. PCOS has not been found to affect the external genitals of newborns, though it can on rare occasions cause *clitoromegaly* (enlargement of the clitoris) in adulthood (Marshall 2001).

The main findings from CAH research regarding psychology are that girls with CAH are more aggressive than their unaffected sisters (Pasterski et al. 2007), show increased male-typical play behaviour (e.g. Berenbaum and Hines 1992), reduced heterosexual orientation (e.g. Hines et al. 2004), better targeting ability in throwing (Hines et al. 2003), and reduced interest in infants (Leveroni and Berenbaum 1998; Mathews et al. 2009). The degree of influence on male-typical play behaviour has been found to relate to the severity of the CAH disorder (e.g. Nordenstrom et al. 2002).

Sample sizes in CAH research are small because the condition is rare. However, the literature on CAH provides a reasonably sound analogue to the kinds of effects of testosterone that might be seen in PCOS, and, indeed, there is some evidence for similar types of effects of testosterone in PCOS as CAH. For example, Manlove et al. (2008) found that women with PCOS reported less female-typical behaviour in childhood, though not at adolescence or adulthood. Agrawal et al. (2004) found a significantly higher prevalence of PCOS and higher testosterone levels in lesbians compared with heterosexual women, but this finding has not been replicated (e.g. De Sutter et al. 2008). Regarding aggression, Elsenbruch et al. (2003) found that women with PCOS were significantly more aggressive than controls, but this difference became statistically non-significant when BMI (body mass index, calculated using metric units as weight divided by height squared) was statistically controlled for. Ingudomnukul et al. (2007) found that PCOS was more common in women with autistic spectrum disorder than healthy controls. However, it should be noted that the difference seen in this study was because PCOS was unusually low in the control group sample (2.7%), and normal rather than high in the autistic spectrum disorder (ASD) group (11.3%). Regarding cognition, women with PCOS have been found to perform less well than controls on verbal fluency, a cognitive task that usually favours women over men (Schattmann and Sherwin 2007), although other cognitive outcomes that often show sex differences (e.g. 3-D mental rotation) are not always found different in PCOS compared to control women (see an interesting discussion of this in Chap. 4 of this book).

The majority of studies of boys with CAH show no difference between subjects and controls. There are two published exceptions: one study found reduced rough and tumble play in boys with CAH (Hines and Kaufman 1994), and another found reduced self-reported male-typical behaviour in boys with CAH (Slijper 1984), but these anomalies in the CAH literature may be caused by the boys' frequent hospitalisation during their first two years of life (Hines 2004). Similarly, effects of PCOS in males are minor compared to consequences for females, and lack much evidence. For example, early baldness has been suggested (Dusková and Stárka 2006) as have raised dehydroepiandrosterone sulphate (DHEAS) and a tendency to insulin resistance (IR) (Sam et al. 2008), but as yet none of these findings have been replicated. However, amongst two relatively large samples of non-PCOS participants a significant relationship has been found between maternal testosterone during pregnancy and gender-role behaviour in the offspring. Hines et al. (2002) found markers of high maternal androgen associated with masculinised gender-role behaviour in female offspring, and Udry et al. (1995) found that gender-typical behaviour was related to hormones from maternal serum only during the second trimester. More research in PCOS is needed, particularly any differences in male children of mothers with PCOS.

Biochemical Aspects of Testosterone

The principal gonadal hormones are testosterone and estradiol. Testosterone is an anabolic steroid and the prototypic hormone of the androgen family of sex hormones. Androgens affect masculine sexual development and function. Testosterone is considered the male sex hormone because the testes predominantly produce testosterone, and testosterone levels are normally about ten times higher in men than in women. Similarly, estradiol is considered the female hormone as the ovaries predominantly produce estrogens, and estradiol levels are usually much higher in women than in men. Testosterone is synthesised from androstenedione and androstenediol, both of which come from DHEA. Testosterone can be synthesised into estradiol or the androgen dihydrotestosterone (DHT), which is roughly three times more potent than testosterone. It is of note that DHEAS is a product of the adrenal glands and a precursor of testosterone; thus, not only is testosterone produced by the gonads (testes and ovaries) but it is also a by-product of androgens from the adrenal glands (androstenedione and DHEAS). It is estimated that in healthy women roughly 25% of testosterone is the result of adrenal androgens (Burger 2002), though the percentage is probably higher in PCOS because the adrenals are hyperresponsive to the stress hormone adrenocorticotropic hormone (ACTH) in PCOS (McKenna and Cunningham 1995; Moran et al. 2004).

Estradiol is the principal estrogenic hormone. The other main estrogen is estrone (E1). Perhaps surprisingly, testosterone is the biochemical precursor of estradiol. Testosterone is converted to estradiol by the enzyme aromatase, and though it has been speculated that a dysfunction in aromatase contributes to the higher testosterone levels seen in PCOS (Xita et al. 2008), we now understand that the impact of AMH on aromatase is to blame (Tata et al. 2018).

Sex hormone binding globulin (SHBG) is the main substance that attaches to sex hormones, and in binding to testosterone and estradiol renders them biologically inert. Its binding affinity is roughly twice as strong for testosterone than for estradiol (Rosner 1991). Thus, higher levels of circulating SHBG will reduce androgenic activity more than estrogenic. Knowledge of binding by SHBG has led to the use of measurements of *free androgens*, for example, the free androgen index (FAI, sometimes known as the free testosterone index, or FTI), which calculates the amount of testosterone that is biologically available in the blood once the amount of bound testosterone has been taken into account. The FAI is often considered a better measure of the androgenic potential in serum than total testosterone. However, the FAI is not always used because the cost and inconvenience of the extra step of measuring SHBG are not always considered to outweigh the benefit of knowing the FAI as opposed to the total testosterone level.

Testosterone has a masculinising effect and can cause females to gain male-typical characteristics or lose female-typical ones. The effects of testosterone can be subdivided roughly into two types: (1) *organisational effects* occur pre- or neonatally and are permanent, and (2) *activational effects* occur after puberty and are reversible. Structural changes in the brain can result from either type of influence.

Three models describe the effects of sex hormones: the gradient model, the classic model, and the multidimensional model. The *gradient model* suggests that the effects of sex hormones are dose-dependent and the level of exposure to a hormone will affect the degree to which masculinisation or feminisation occurs. The *classic model* suggests that testosterone causes masculinisation and reduces feminisation, and absence of testosterone causes feminisation and reduces masculinisation, and there is a lot of evidence to support this model (Pfaff et al. 2002). For example, all mammalian fetuses will develop as phenotypic females unless the Y chromosome (called SRY) causes the gonads to differentiate as testes and produce testosterone (Wilson et al. 1981). Prenatal exposure to testosterone can alter brain structure, for example, creating a male-typical development of aromatase-expressing neurons in the sexually dimorphic nucleus of female sheep (Roselli et al. 2007). The *multidimensional model* (see below) allows for expansion beyond the gradient and classic models.

Although estrogens are necessary for female-typical maturation and function in adulthood, they appear to have little or no role in promoting female development of the fetus. However, active feminisation of behaviour by estrogens occurs at other times; for example, Dunlap et al. (1978) found that in rats near puberty, ovarian hormones make permanent some aspects of female-typical sexual behaviour.

There is also evidence that there are critical or sensitive periods for the influence of testosterone on development in animals, though evidence in humans is limited (principally due to ethical constraints in research in this area). For example, female mammals exposed to testosterone during pre- or neonatal critical periods show increased sexual behaviour in adulthood towards females and reduced sexual responding to males; likewise, depriving males of testosterone during pre- or neonatal critical periods results in reduced male-typical and increased female-typical sexual behaviour in adulthood (Goy and McEwen 1980; Beach 1975).

There is evidence that masculinisation and feminisation are separate dimensions, and the simple idea of testosterone causing male-typical development and the absence of testosterone causing female-typical development is an oversimplification; there are examples in rodents that demonstrate that in many cases testosterone needs to be converted to estradiol before acting on the estradiol receptors to create male-typical neural and behavioural development (McCarthy 2008). However, it is likely that the type of pathway will differ by species and by type of behaviour, and Hines (2009) suggests this sexual differentiation is best understood by a *multidimensional model* that resolves apparent contradictions between earlier models.

It can be difficult to differentiate between the effect of nature and the postnatal environment, especially when studying human behaviour. Traditionally, the literature on sex difference uses the term 'gender' to identify sex differences with cultural causes (e.g. the wearing of trousers rather than skirts) and the term 'sex' for difference due to biology (e.g. having internal ovaries rather than external testes). However, in many cases it is very difficult to establish whether a sex difference is mainly due to nature, nurture, or is some roughly equal combination of both. For this reason some authors use the terms sex and gender interchangeably.

The Role of Insulin in Androgen Production

Insulin causes androgen production in the ovaries (Yen 1991), and there is a positive correlation between testosterone and insulin levels in women with PCOS (Buffington et al. 1991). Indeed, insulin and testosterone are in a cyclical relationship: insulin promotes testosterone, testosterone promotes visceral fat and insulin resistance, and this elevates insulin levels (Stanley and Misra 2008).

Insulin resistance can be genetic or the result of a lifestyle characterised by a lack of exercise, high-carbohydrate diet, and stress. Insulin resistance is caused when the number of insulin receptors on cell walls is reduced, and in PCOS this reduction can be up to 75% (reduced from roughly 20,000 receptors to 5000 receptors). This means that the ability of serum glucose (blood sugar) to enter the cell to be converted to energy is reduced, and must instead remain in the bloodstream until converted by the liver into fat. The accumulation of fat leads to obesity, which in itself can contribute to PCOS. In women, carrying weight on the stomach rather than hips is known as central (or android) obesity, and is related to elevated androgen levels. Although insulin resistance also occurs in non-obese women (Dunaif et al. 1989), non-diabetic women with central obesity typically have elevated androgens, insulin resistance, and hyperinsulinemia (elevated blood insulin levels) (Kissebah et al. 1982). It seems likely then that insulin plays an important role in PCOS, though whether it is more important than testosterone is open to debate (Azziz et al. 2008) and may depend on the PCOS phenotype in question (see above) or the level at which etiology is being considered.

Drug treatment of PCOS usually aims to reduce testosterone levels, either indirectly by using the insulin sensitiser metformin or directly by using anti-androgens or contraceptives that have an anti-androgenic effect (e.g. Dianette). Hunter and Sterrett (2000) suggest that metformin reduces testosterone levels and restores normal menstrual cyclicity. Pasquali et al. (2000) found that metformin decreased testosterone levels in women with PCOS, and that both women with PCOS and healthy controls treated with metformin experienced a reduction in their BMI. Despite insulin resistance often being seen in PCOS, the ovaries remain sensitive to insulin; there is as yet no explanation for this phenomenon (Diamanti-Kandarkis et al. 2008).

Concluding Comments for the Introduction

As can be seen, PCOS is a complex condition and completing our knowledge of even the most basic aspects of it—the causes and the most reliable treatments—still requires a great deal of research. It also remains to be seen whether psychological factors in PCOS are directly caused by testosterone (due to prenatal organisation, or activation by circulating testosterone—see Chap. 7), or other factors such as blood glucose fluctuations (see Chap. 5), or are simply caused by the stress of having PCOS symptoms (see Chap. 2). The remainder of this book describes studies that attempt to address these issues, and, based on these findings, suggests new hypotheses to be explored.

References

Abbott, D. H., Eisner, J. R., Goodfriend, T., Medley, R. D., Peterson, E. J., Colman, R. J., ... Dumesic, D. A. (2002, June 19–22). *Leptin and total free fatty acids are elevated in the circulation of prenatally androgenized female rhesus monkeys*. Abstract P2–329. 84th Annual Meeting of The Endocrine Society, San Francisco, CA.

Acién, P., Quereda, F., Matallín, P., Villarroya, E., López-Fernández, J. A., Acién, M., … Alfayate, R. (1999). Insulin, androgens, and obesity in women with and without polycystic ovary syndrome: A heterogeneous group of disorders. *Fertility and Sterility, 72*(1), 32–40.

Agrawal, R., Sharma, S., Bekir, J., Conway, G., Bailey, J., Balen, A. H., & Prelevic, G. (2004). Prevalence of polycystic ovaries and polycystic ovary syndrome in lesbian women compared with heterosexual women. *Fertility and Sterility, 82*, 1352–1357.

Anderson, S. A., Barry, J. A., & Hardiman, P. J. (2014). Risk of coronary heart disease and risk of stroke in women with polycystic ovary syndrome: A systematic review and meta-analysis. *International Journal of Cardiology, 176*(2), 486–487.

Astapova, O., Minor, B. M., & Hammes, S. R. (2019). Physiological and pathological androgen actions in the ovary. *Endocrinology, 160*(5), 1166–1174.

Azziz, R. (2006). Controversy in clinical endocrinology: Diagnosis of polycystic ovarian syndrome: The Rotterdam criteria are premature. *The Journal of Clinical Endocrinology and Metabolism, 9*, 781–785.

Azziz, R. (2014). Polycystic ovary syndrome: What's in a name? *The Journal of Clinical Endocrinology and Metabolism, 99*(4), 1142–1145.

Azziz, R., Carmina, E., Dewailly, D., Diamanti-Kandarakis, E., Escobar-Morreale, H. F., Futterweit, W., … Androgen Excess Society. (2006). Position statement: Criteria for defining polycystic ovary syndrome as a predominantly hyperandrogenic syndrome: An Androgen Excess Society guideline. *The Journal of Clinical Endocrinology and Metabolism, 91*, 4237–4245. https://doi.org/10.1210/jc.2006-0178.

Azziz, R., Carmina, E., Dewailly, D., Diamanti-Kandarakis, E., Escobar-Morreale, H. F., Futterweit, W., … (Task Force on the Phenotype of the Polycystic Ovary Syndrome of The Androgen Excess and PCOS Society). (2008). The Androgen Excess and PCOS Society criteria for the polycystic ovary syndrome: The complete task force report. *Fertility and Sterility, 91*, 456–488.

Azziz, R., Carmina, E., Dewailly, D., Diamanti-Kandarakis, E., Escobar-Morreale, H. F., Futterweit, W., … Witchel, S. F. (2009). The androgen excess and PCOS society criteria for the polycystic ovary syndrome: The complete task force report. *Fertility and Sterility, 91*(2), 456–488.

Azziz, R., Marin, C., Hoq, L., Badamgarav, E., & Song, P. (2005). Health care-related economic burden of the polycystic ovary syndrome during the reproductive life span. *The Journal of Clinical Endocrinology & Metabolism, 90*(8), 4650–4658.

Barclay, L., & Murata, P. (2006, October). Obese premenopausal women are at high risk for PCOS. *Medscape Today*. Retrieved October 16, 2008, from http://www.medscape.com/viewarticle/546731.

Barker, D. J. (2004). The developmental origins of chronic adult disease. *Acta Paediatrica Supplement, 93*, 26–33.

Barrett, E. S., Hoeger, K. M., Sathyanarayana, S., Abbott, D. H., Redmon, J. B., Nguyen, R. H. N., & Swan, S. H. (2018). Anogenital distance in newborn daughters of women with polycystic ovary syndrome indicates fetal testosterone exposure. *Journal of Developmental Origins of Health and Disease, 9*(3), 307–314.

Barry, J. A., Kay, A. R., Navaratnarajah, R., Iqbal, S., Bamfo, J. E. A. K., David, A. L., … Hardiman, P. J. (2010). Umbilical vein testosterone in female infants born to mothers with polycystic ovary syndrome is elevated to male levels. *Journal of Obstetrics and Gynaecology, 30*(5), 444–446.

Barry, J. A., Hardiman, P. J., Saxby, B. K., & Kuczmierczyk, A. (2011). Testosterone and mood dysfunction in women with polycystic ovarian syndrome compared to subfertile controls. *Journal of Psychosomatic Obstetrics and Gynecology, 32*(2), 104–111.

Barry, J. A., Azizia, M. M., & Hardiman, P. J. (2014). Risk of endometrial, ovarian and breast cancer in women with polycystic ovary syndrome: A systematic review and meta-analysis. *Human Reproduction Update, 20*(5), 748–758.

Barry, J. A., & Owens, R. (2019). From fetuses to boys to men: The impact of testosterone on male lifespan development. In *The Palgrave handbook of male psychology and mental health* (pp. 3–24). Cham: Palgrave Macmillan.

Beach, F. A. (1975). Hormonal modification of sexually dimorphic behavior. *Psychoneuroendocrinology, 1*, 3–23.

Berenbaum, S. A., & Hines, M. (1992). Early androgens are related to childhood sex-typed toy preferences. *Psychological Science, 3*, 203–206.

Buffington, C. K., Givens, J. R., & Kitabchi, A. E. (1991). Opposing actions of dehydroepiandrosterone and testosterone on insulin sensitivity. In vivo and in vitro studies of hyperandrogenic females. *Diabetes, 40*, 693–700.

Burger, H. G. (2002). Androgen production in women. *Fertility and Sterility, 77*, S3–S5.

Busby, M., & Simpson, L. (2019, April). *Perceptions of coping with the long-term consequences of polycystic ovary syndrome at different stages of the menopausal transition*. Poster session presented at the meeting of the British Psychological Society NI Branch 2019 Annual Conference, Belfast, NI. https://doi.org/10.13140/RG.2.2.35669.88803.

Cesta, C. E., Månsson, M., Palm, C., Lichtenstein, P., Iliadou, A. N., & Landén, M. (2016). Polycystic ovary syndrome and psychiatric disorders: Co-morbidity and heritability in a nationwide Swedish cohort. *Psychoneuroendocrinology, 73*, 196–203.

Dapas, M., Sisk, R., Legro, R. S., Urbanek, M., Dunaif, A., & Hayes, M. G. (2019). Family-based quantitative trait meta-analysis implicates rare noncoding variants in DENND1A in polycystic ovary syndrome. *The Journal of Clinical Endocrinology & Metabolism, 104*(9), 3835–3850.

Day, F., Karaderi, T., Jones, M. R., Meun, C., He, C., Drong, A., … Magi, R. (2018). Large-scale genome-wide meta-analysis of polycystic ovary syndrome suggests shared genetic architecture for different diagnosis criteria. *PLoS Genetics, 14*(12), e1007813.

De Sutter, P., Dutré, T. I. N. E. K. E., Meerschaut, F. V., Stuyver, I., Van Maele, G. E. O. R. G. E. S., & Dhont, M. (2008). PCOS in lesbian and heterosexual women treated with artificial donor insemination. *Reproductive Biomedicine Online, 17*(3), 398–402.

Dhurandhar, N. V., Kulkarni, P. R., Ajinkya, S. M., Sherikar, A. A., & Atkinson, R. L. (1997). Association of adenovirus infection with human obesity. *Obesity Research, 5*, 464–469.

Dhurandhar, N. V., Whigham, L. D., Abbott, D. H., Schultz-Darken, N. J., Israel, B. A., Bradley, S. M., … Atkinson, R. L. (2002). Human adenovirus Ad-36 promotes weight gain in male rhesus and marmoset monkeys. *The Journal of Nutrition, 132*, 3155–3160.

Diamanti-Kandarakis, E., Kandarakis, H., & Legro, R. S. (2006). The role of genes and environment in the etiology of PCOS. *Endocrine, 30*, 19–26.

Diamanti-Kandarakis, E., Christakou, C., Palioura, E., Kandaraki, E., & Livadas, S. (2008). Does polycystic ovary syndrome start in childhood? *Pediatric Endocrinology Reviews, 5*, 904–911.

Ding, T., Hardiman, P. J., Petersen, I., & Baio, G. (2018). Incidence and prevalence of diabetes and cost of illness analysis of polycystic ovary syndrome: A Bayesian modelling study. *Human Reproduction, 33*(7), 1299–1306.

Dumesic, D. A., Abbott, D. H., & Padmanabhan, V. (2007). Polycystic ovary syndrome and its developmental origins. *Reviews in Endocrine & Metabolic Disorders, 8*(2), 127–141.

Dunaif, A., & Fauser, B. C. (2013). Renaming PCOS—A two-state solution. *The Journal of Clinical Endocrinology & Metabolism, 98*(11), 4325–4328.

Dunaif, A., & Thomas, A. (2001). Current concepts in the polycystic ovary syndrome. *Annual Review of Medicine, 52*, 401–419.

Dunaif, A., Segal, K. R., Futterweit, W., & Dobrjansky, A. (1989). Profound peripheral insulin resistance, independent of obesity, in polycystic ovary syndrome. *Diabetes, 38*, 1165–1174.

Dunlap, J. L., Gerall, A. A., & Carlton, S. F. (1978). Evaluation of prenatal androgen and ovarian secretions on receptivity in female and male rats. *Journal of Comparative and Physiological Psychology, 92*, 280–288.

Dusková, M., & Stárka, L. (2006). The existence of a male equivalent of the polycystic ovary syndrome—The present state of the issue. *Prague Medical Report, 107*, 17–25.

Eggers, S., & Kirchengast, S. (2001). The polycystic ovary syndrome—A medical condition but also an important psychosocial problem. *Collegium Antropologicum, 25*, 673–685.

Eggers, S., Hashimoto, D. M., & Kirchengast, S. (2007). An evolutionary approach to explain the high frequency of the polycystic ovary syndrome (PCOS). *Anthropologischer Anzeiger, 65*, 169–179.

Elsenbruch, S., Hahn, S., Kowalsky, D., Offner, A. H., Schedlowski, M., Mann, K., & Janssen, O. E. (2003). Quality of life, psychosocial well-being, and sexual satisfaction in women with polycystic ovary syndrome. *The Journal of Clinical Endocrinology and Metabolism, 88*, 5801–5807.

Escobar-Morreale, H. F. (2018). Polycystic ovary syndrome: Definition, aetiology, diagnosis and treatment. *Nature Reviews. Endocrinology, 14*(5), 270–284.

Escobar-Morreale, H. F., Luque-Ramírez, M., & San Millán, J. L. (2005). The molecular-genetic basis of functional hyperandrogenism and the polycystic ovary syndrome. *Endocrine Reviews, 26*, 251–282.

Farrell, K., & Antoni, M. H. (2010). Insulin resistance, obesity, inflammation, and depression in polycystic ovary syndrome: Biobehavioral mechanisms and interventions. *Fertility and Sterility, 94*(5), 1565–1574.

Filippou, P., & Homburg, R. (2017). Is foetal hyperexposure to androgens a cause of PCOS? *Human Reproduction Update, 23*(4), 421–432.

Forest, M. G., Bétuel, H., Couillin, P., & Boué, A. (1981). Prenatal diagnosis of congenital adrenal hyperplasia (CAH) due to 21-hydroxylase deficiency by steroid analysis in the amniotic fluid of mid-pregnancy: Comparison with HLA typing in 17 pregnancies at risk for CAH. *Prenatal Diagnosis, 1*, 197–207.

Franceschi, R., Gaudino, R., Marcolongo, A., Chiara Gallo, M., Rossi, L., Antoniazzi, F., & Tatò, L. (2009). Prevalence of polycystic ovary syndrome in young women who had idiopathic central precocious puberty. *Fertility and Sterility, 93*(4), 1185–1191. In Press, Corrected Proof, Available online 9 January 2009.

Franks, S. (2008). Polycystic ovary syndrome in adolescents. *International Journal of Obesity, 32*, 1035–1041.

Franks, S., Mccarthy, M. I., & Hardy, K. (2006). Development of polycystic ovary syndrome: Involvement of genetic and environmental factors. *International Journal of Andrology, 29*(1), 278–285.

Gallinelli, A., Matteo, M. L., Volpe, A., & Facchinetti, F. (2000). Autonomic and neuroendocrine responses to stress in patients with functional hypothalamic secondary amenorrhea. *Fertility and Sterility, 73*, 812–816.

Gelis, J. (1989). The secret of birth. *Histoire des Sciences Médicales, 23*, 109–114.

Genton, P., Bauer, J., Duncan, S., Taylor, A. E., Balen, A. H., Eberle, A., … Sauer, M. V. (2001). On the association between valproate and polycystic ovary syndrome. *Epilepsia, 42*, 295–304.

Gersh, F., & Parella, A. (2018). *PCOS SOS. A gynecologist's lifeline to naturally restore your rhythms, hormones, and happiness.* Irvine: Integrative Medical Group.

Glueck, C. J., Goldenberg, N., Wang, P., Loftspring, M., & Sherman, A. (2004). Metformin during pregnancy reduces insulin, insulin resistance, insulin secretion, weight, testosterone and development of gestational diabetes: Prospective longitudinal assessment of women with polycystic ovary syndrome from preconception throughout pregnancy. *Human Reproduction, 19*, 510–521.

Gore, A. C., Chappell, V. A., Fenton, S. E., Flaws, J. A., Nadal, A., Prins, G. S., … Zoeller, R. T. (2015). EDC-2: The endocrine society's second scientific statement on endocrine-disrupting chemicals. *Endocrine Reviews, 36*(6), E1–E150.

Gougeon, A. (1996). Regulation of ovarian follicular development in primates: Facts and hypotheses. *Endocrine Reviews, 17*(2), 121–155.

Goy, R. W., & McEwen, B. S. (1980). *Sexual differentiation of the brain.* Cambridge, MA: MIT Press.

Goyal, M., & Dawood, A. S. (2017). Debates regarding lean patients with polycystic ovary syndrome: A narrative review. *Journal of Human Reproductive Sciences, 10*(3), 154.

Hamilton, W. G. (1963). The evolution of altruistic behavior. *American Naturalist, 97*, 354–356.

Hamilton, W. G. (1964a). The genetical evolution of social behavior. I. *Journal of Theoretical Biology, 7*, 1–16.

Hamilton, W. G. (1964b). The genetical evolution of social behaviour. II. *Journal of Theoretical Biology, 7*, 17–27.

Harris, J. A., Vernon, P. A., & Boomsma, D. I. (1998). The heritability of testosterone: A study of Dutch adolescent twins and their parents. *Behavior
Genetics, 28*, 165–171.

Hawkes, K., O'Connell, J. F., Jones, N. G., Alvarez, H., & Charnov, E. L.
(1998). Grandmothering, menopause, and the evolution of human life histo-
ries. *Proceedings of the National Academy of Sciences, 95*, 1336–1339.

Hines, M. (2002). Sexual differentiation of human brain and behaviour. In
D. Pfaff, A. P. Arnold, A. M. Etgen, S. E. Fahrbach, & R. T. Rubin (Eds.),
Hormones, brain and behavior (Vol. 4, pp. 425–462). New York:
Academic Press.

Hines, M. (2009). Gonadal hormones and sexual differentiation of human
brain and behavior. In P. D. W. Hormones (Ed.), *Brain and Behavior* (2nd
ed., pp. 1869–1909). New York: Academic Press.

Hines, M., & Kaufman, F. R. (1994). Androgen and the development of human
sex-typical behavior: Rough-and-tumble play and sex of preferred playmates
in children with congenital adrenal hyperplasia (CAH). *Child Development,
65*(4), 1042–1053.

Hines, M., Brook, C., & Conway, G. S. (2004). Androgen and psychosexual
development: Core gender identity, sexual orientation and recalled childhood gender role behavior in women and men with congenital adrenal
hyperplasia (CAH). *Journal of Sex Research, 41*, 1–7.

Hines, M., Fane, B. A., Pasterski, V. L., Mathews, G. A., Conway, G. S., &
Brook, C. (2003). Spatial abilities following prenatal androgen abnormality:
Targeting and mental rotations performance in individuals with congenital
adrenal hyperplasia. *Psychoneuroendocrinology, 28*(8), 1010–1026.

Homburg, R., & Crawford, G. (2014). The role of AMH in anovulation associated with PCOS: A hypothesis. *Human Reproduction, 29*, 1117–1121.

Hong, Y., Gagnon, J., Rice, T., Pérusse, L., Leon, A. S., Skinner, J. S., … Rao,
D. C. (2001). Familial resemblance for free androgens and androgen gluc-
uronides in sedentary black and white individuals: The HERITAGE Family
Study. Health, Risk Factors, Exercise Training and Genetics. *The Journal of
Endocrinology, 70*, 485–492.

Hrdy, S. B. (1999). *Mother nature*. Berlin: Verlag.

Hu, S., Leonard, A., Seifalian, A., & Hardiman, P. (2007). Vascular dysfunction
during pregnancy in women with polycystic ovary syndrome. *Human
Reproduction, 22*, 1532–1539.

Hunter, M. H., & Sterrett, J. J. (2000). Polycystic ovary syndrome: It's not just
infertility. *American Family Physician, 62*, 1079–1088.

Ingudomnukul, E., Baron-Cohen, S., Wheelwright, S., & Knickmeyer, R. (2007). Elevated rates of testosterone-related disorders in women with autism spectrum conditions. *Hormones and Behavior, 51*, 597–604.

Iniguez, G., Ong, K., Bazaes, R., Avila, A., Salazar, T., Dunger, D., & Mericq, V. (2006). Longitudinal changes in insulin-like growth factor-I, insulin sensitivity, and secretion from birth to age three years in small-for-gestational-age children. *The Journal of Clinical Endocrinology & Metabolism, 91*(11), 4645–4649.

Isojärvi, J. I., Rättyä, J., Myllylä, V. V., Knip, M., Koivunen, R., Pakarinen, A. J., ... Tapanainen, J. S. (1998). Valproate, lamotrigine, and insulin-mediated risks in women with epilepsy. *Annals of Neurology, 43*(4), 446–451.

Jahanfar, S., Maleki, H., Mosavi, A. R., & Jahanfar, M. (2004). Leptin and its association with polycystic ovary syndrome: A twin study. *Gynecological Endocrinology, 18*, 327–334.

Kahsar-Miller, M. D., Nixon, C., Boots, L. R., Go, R. C., & Azziz, R. (2001). Prevalence of polycystic ovary syndrome (PCOS) in first-degree relatives of patients with PCOS. *Fertility and Sterility, 75*, 53–58.

Kandaraki, E., Chatzigeorgiou, A., Livadas, S., Palioura, E., Economou, F., Koutsilieris, M., ... Diamanti-Kandarakis, E. (2011). Endocrine disruptors and polycystic ovary syndrome (PCOS): Elevated serum levels of bisphenol A in women with PCOS. *The Journal of Clinical Endocrinology & Metabolism, 96*(3), E480–E484.

Keski-Rahkonen, A., Bulik, C. M., Pietiläinen, K. H., Rose, R. J., Kaprio, J., & Rissanen, A. (2007). Eating styles, overweight and obesity in young adult twins. *European Journal of Clinical Nutrition, 61*, 822–829.

Kissebah, A. H., Vydelingum, N., Murray, R., Evans, D. J., Hartz, A. J., Kalkhoff, R. K., & Adams, P. W. (1982). Relation of body fat distribution to metabolic complications of obesity. *Clinics in Endocrinology and Metabolism, 54*, 254–260.

Kitzinger, C., & Willmott, J. (2002). 'The thief of womanhood': Women's experience of polycystic ovarian syndrome. *Social Science & Medicine, 54*, 349–361.

Kondoh, Y., Uemura, T., Ishikawa, M., Yokoi, N., & Hirahara, F. (1999). Classification of polycystic ovary syndrome into three types according to response to human corticotropin-releasing hormone. *Fertility and Sterility, 72*, 15–20.

Lambertini, L., Saul, S. R., Copperman, A. B., Hammerstad, S. S., Yi, Z., Zhang, W., ... Kase, N. (2017). Intrauterine reprogramming of the polycystic ovary syndrome: Evidence from a pilot study of cord blood global methylation analysis. *Frontiers in Endocrinology, 8*, 352.

Lazurova, Z., Figurova, J., Hubkova, B., & Lazurova, I. (2018, May). Relationship of urinary bisphenol A to metabolic and hormonal profile in PCOS women. In *20th European Congress of Endocrinology* (Vol. 56). Bristol: BioScientifica.

Legro, R. S., Driscoll, D., Strauss, J. F., Fox, J., & Dunaif, A. (1998). Evidence for a genetic basis for hyperandrogenemia in polycystic ovary syndrome. *Proceedings of the National Academy of Sciences, 95*(25), 14956–14960.

Leveroni, C. L., & Berenbaum, S. A. (1998). Early androgen effects on interest in infants: Evidence from children with congenital adrenal hyperplasia. *Developmental Neuropsychology, 14*, 321–340.

Li, T. T., Xu, L. Z., Chen, Y. H., Deng, H. M., Liang, C. Y., Liu, Y., ... Han, D. W. (2011). Effects of eight environmental endocrine disruptors on insulin resistance in patients with polycystic ovary syndrome: A preliminary investigation. *Nan fang yi ke da xue xue bao= Journal of Southern Medical University, 31*(10), 1753–1756.

Manikkam, M., Crespi, E. J., Doop, D. D., Herkimer, C., Lee, J. S., Yu, S., ... Padmanabhan, V. (2004). Fetal programming: Prenatal testosterone excess leads to fetal growth retardation and postnatal catch-up growth in sheep. *Endocrinology, 145*, 790–798.

Manlove, H. A., Guillermo, C., & Gray, P. B. (2008). Do women with polycystic ovary syndrome (PCOS) report differences in sex-typed behavior as children and adolescents?: Results of a pilot study. *Annals of Human Biology, 35*, 584–595.

Marshall, K. (2001). Polycystic ovary syndrome: Clinical considerations. *Alternative Medicine Review, 6*, 272–292.

Mathews, G. A., Fane, B. A., Conway, G. S., Brook, C. G., & Hines, M. (2009). Personality and congenital adrenal hyperplasia: Possible effects of prenatal androgen exposure. *Hormones and Behavior, 55*, 285–291.

McCarthy, M. M. (2008). Estradiol and the developing brain. *Physiological Reviews, 88*, 91–134.

McKenna, T. J., & Cunningham, S. K. (1995). Adrenal androgen production in polycystic ovary syndrome. *European Journal of Endocrinology, 133*, 383–389.

Miazgowski, T., Martopullo, I., Widecka, J., Miazgowski, B., & Brodowska, A. (2019). National and regional trends in the prevalence of polycystic ovary syndrome since 1990 within Europe: The modeled estimates from the Global Burden of Disease Study 2016. *Archives of Medical Science, 15*(1). https://doi.org/10.5114/aoms.2019.87112.

Miller, W. L., & Levine, L. S. (1987). Molecular and clinical advances in congenital adrenal hyperplasia. *The Journal of Pediatrics, 111*, 1–17.

Moran, L. J., Brinkworth, G., Noakes, M., & Norman, R. J. (2006). Effects of lifestyle modification in polycystic ovarian syndrome. *Reproductive Biomedicine Online, 12*, 569–578.

Moran, C., Reyna, R., Boots, L. S., & Azziz, R. (2004). Adrenocortical hyper-responsiveness to corticotropin in polycystic ovary syndrome patients with adrenal androgen excess. *Fertility and Sterility, 81*(1), 126–131.

Nestler, J. E. (1990). Insulin-like growth factor II is a potent inhibitor of the aromatase activity of human placental cytotrophoblasts. *Endocrinology, 127*, 2064–2070.

Nordenstrom, A., Servin, A., Bohlin, G., Larsson, A., & Wedell, A. (2002). Sex-typed toy play behavior correlates with the degree of prenatal androgen exposure assessed by CYP21 genotype in girls with congenital adrenal hyperplasia. *Journal of Clinical Endocrinology and Metabolism, 87*, 5119–5124.

Norman, R. J., Dewailly, D., Legro, R. S., & Hickey, T. E. (2007). Polycystic ovary syndrome. *Lancet, 370*, 685–697.

Pasquali, R., Gambineri, A., Biscotti, D., Vicennati, V., Gagliardi, L., Colitta, D., ... Morselli-Labate, A. M. (2000). Effect of long-term treatment with metformin added to hypocaloric diet on body composition, fat distribution, and androgen and insulin levels in abdominally obese women with and without the polycystic ovary syndrome. *The Journal of Clinical Endocrinology & Metabolism, 85*(8), 2767–2774.

Pasterski, V., Hindmarsh, P., Geffner, M., Brook, C., Brain, C., & Hines, M. (2007). Increased aggression and activity level in 3- to 11-year-old girls with congenital adrenal hyperplasia (CAH). *Hormones and Behavior, 52*, 368–374.

Pellatt, L., Rice, S., & Mason, H. D. (2010). Anti-Müllerian hormone and polycystic ovary syndrome: A mountain too high? *Reproduction, 139*, 825–833.

Pfaff, D., Arnold, A.P., Etgen, A.M., Fahrbach, S.E., & Rubin, R.T. (Eds.). (2002). *Hormones, brain and behavior* (Vol. 4, pp. 425–462). New York: Academic Press.

Resko, J. A., Buhl, A. E., & Phoenix, C. H. (1987). Treatment of pregnant rhesus macaques with testosterone propionate: Observations on its fate in the fetus. *Biology of Reproduction, 37*, 1185–1191.

Resko, J. A., & Ellinwood, W. E. (1984). Sexual differentiation of testosterone he brain of primates. In M. Serio, M. Motta, M. Zanisi, & L. Martini (Eds.), *Sexual differentiation: Basic and clinical aspects* (pp. 169–181). New York: Raven Press.

Roselli, C. E., Stadelman, H., Reeve, R., Bishop, C. V., & Stormshak, F. (2007). The ovine sexually dimorphic nucleus of the medial preoptic area is organized prenatally by testosterone. *Endocrinology, 148*, 4450–4457.

Rosner, W. (1991). Plasma steroid binding proteins. *Endocrinology and Metabolism Clinics of North America, 20*, 697–720.

Sam, S. (2007). Obesity and polycystic ovary syndrome. *Obesity Management, 3*, 69–73.

Sam, S., Coviello, A. D., Sung, Y. A., Legro, R. S., & Dunaif, A. (2008). Metabolic phenotype in the brothers of women with polycystic ovary syndrome. *Diabetes Care, 31*(6), 1237–1241.

Schattmann, L., & Sherwin, B. B. (2007). Testosterone levels and cognitive functioning in women with polycystic ovary syndrome and in healthy young women. *Hormones and Behavior, 51*, 587–596.

Schenker, J. G. (2000). Women's reproductive health: Monotheistic religious perspectives. *International Journal of Gynaecology and Obstetrics, 70*, 77–86.

Shaw, L. M., & Elton, S. (2008). Polycystic ovary syndrome: A transgenerational evolutionary adaptation. *BJOG, 115*, 144–148.

Slijper, F. M. (1984). Androgens and gender role behaviour in girls with congenital adrenal hyperplasia (CAH). In *Progress in brain research* (Vol. 61, pp. 417–422). Amsterdam: Elsevier.

Smail, P. J., Reyes, F. I., Winter, J. S. D., & Faiman, C. (1981). The fetal hormonal environment and its effect on the morphogenesis of the genital system. In S. J. Kogan & E. S. E. Hafez (Eds.), *Pediatric andrology* (pp. 9–19). The Hague: Martinus Nijhoff.

Stanley, T., & Misra, M. (2008). Polycystic ovary syndrome in obese adolescents. *Current Opinion in Endocrinology, Diabetes, and Obesity, 15*, 30–36.

Sultan, C., & Paris, F. (2008). Clinical expression of polycystic ovary syndrome in adolescent girls. *Fertility and Sterility, 86*(Suppl 1), S6.

Szydlarska, D., Machaj, M., & Jakimiuk, A. (2017). History of discovery of polycystic ovary syndrome. *Advances in Clinical and Experimental Medicine, 26*(3), 555–558.

Tata, B., Mimouni, N. E. H., Barbotin, A. L., Malone, S. A., Loyens, A., Pigny, P., ... Dal Bello, F. (2018). Elevated prenatal anti-Müllerian hormone reprograms the fetus and induces polycystic ovary syndrome in adulthood. *Nature Medicine, 24*(6), 834.

The Rotterdam ESHRE/ASRM—Sponsored PCOS consensus workshop group. Revised 2003 consensus on diagnostic criteria and long-term health risks related to polycystic ovary syndrome (PCOS). *Hum Reprod, 19*, 41–47.

Tsilchorozidou, T., Overton, C., & Conway, G. S. (2004). The pathophysiology of polycystic ovary syndrome. *Clinical Endocrinology, 60*(1), 1–17.

Udry, J. R., Morris, N. M., & Kovenock, J. (1995). Androgen effects on women's gendered behaviour. *Journal of Biosocial Science, 27*(3), 359–368.

Vanky, E., Salvesen, K. A., Heimstad, R., Fougner, K. J., Romundstad, P., & Carlsen, S. M. (2004). Metformin reduces pregnancy complications without affecting androgen levels in pregnant polycystic ovary syndrome women: Results of a randomized study. *Human Reproduction, 19*, 1734–1740.

Vink, J. M., Sadrzadeh, S., Lambalk, C. B., & Boomsma, D. I. (2006). Heritability of polycystic ovary syndrome in a Dutch twin-family study. *The Journal of Clinical Endocrinology and Metabolism, 91*, 2100–2104.

Williamson, K., Gunn, A. J., Johnson, N., & Milsom, S. R. (2001). The impact of ethnicity on the presentation of polycystic ovarian syndrome. *Australian and New Zealand Journal of Obstetrics and Gynaecology, 41*(2), 202–206.

Wilson, J. D., George, F. W., & Griffin, J. E. (1981). The hormonal control of sexual development. *Science, 211*, 1278–1284.

Xita, I., Georgiou, L., Lazaros, V., Psofaki, G. K., & Tsatsoulis, A. (2008). The synergistic effect of sex hormone-binding globulin and aromatase genes on polycystic ovary syndrome phenotype. *European Journal of Endocrinology, 158*, 861–865.

Yen, S. S. C. (1991). Chronic anovulation caused by peripheral report. J. Clin. Psychiatry 61, 173–178. Endocrine disorders. In S. S. C. Yen & R. B. Jaffe (Eds.), *Reproductive endocrinology: Physiology, pathophysiology and clinical management* (3rd ed., pp. 576–630). Philadelphia: W.B. Saunders.

Yilmaz, B., Vellanki, P., Ata, B., & Yildiz, B. O. (2018). Metabolic syndrome, hypertension, and hyperlipidemia in mothers, fathers, sisters, and brothers of women with polycystic ovary syndrome: A systematic review and meta-analysis. *Fertility and Sterility, 109*(2), 356–364.

Zawadski, J. K., & Dunaif, A. (1992). Diagnostic criteria for polycystic ovary syndrome; towards a rational approach. In A. Dunaif, J. R. Givens, & F. Haseltine (Eds.), *Polycystic ovary syndrome* (pp. 377–384). Boston: Blackwell Scientific.

2

Depression in Polycystic Ovary Syndrome

Abstract The psychological issue related to in polycystic ovary syndrome (PCOS) that receives most attention is depression. This chapter explores the causes of depression, examining how much the various symptoms of PCOS (fertility issues, body hair, etc.) contribute to depression in PCOS. This chapter also reassesses some of the research on this topic. Improvements to how we (myself included) research the psychological aspects of PCOS are discussed.

Keywords Depression • Obesity • Hirsutism • Suicide • Methodology

Introduction

In one of the first studies of the psychological aspects of polycystic ovary syndrome (PCOS) Monzani et al. (1994) found that 23 PCOS patients had significantly higher levels of anxiety and depression (measured on the Crown-Crisp Experiential Index) than 20 age-matched healthy control women. Research since then has very often found evidence for greater depression and anxiety in women with PCOS than controls or normative

© The Author(s) 2019
J. A. Barry, *Psychological Aspects of Polycystic Ovary Syndrome*,
https://doi.org/10.1007/978-3-030-30290-0_2

population levels, as confirmed by several meta-analyses (e.g. Barry et al. 2011a; Cooney et al. 2017).

Although in this chapter we will see that the evidence suggests that depression in PCOS is caused mainly by the distressing symptoms of PCOS, healthcare professionals should always be alert to the possibility that for each individual, other factors might be the cause of depression. This might include biopsychological factors (e.g. related to insulin resistance, discussed in Chap. 5), but also more everyday reasons. For example, a woman with PCOS might be depressed about her symptoms, but be more depressed about problems she is experiencing at the workplace that are completely unrelated to PCOS. Thus, the person should always be treated holistically, not simply as a generic case of PCOS.

The finding of higher depression and anxiety has been replicated many times, yet it is not generally recognised that PCOS is an at-risk population for these conditions. There are signs that this is changing; for example, in Australia several years ago the Endocrine Society recommended that women with PCOS be routinely screened for depression and anxiety (Teede et al. 2011), but this practice remains uncommon elsewhere in the world.

Anxiety and depression often co-occur. Of the two, depression is more commonly assessed, and in research where depression is assessed in PCOS, anxiety is also measured in about 60% of these studies (Cooney et al. 2017). They are sometimes measured using the same instrument, most commonly the Hospital Anxiety and Depression Scale (HADS; Zigmond and Snaith 1983).

In this book anxiety and depression are discussed in different chapters because the underlying cause of each is likely to be different (see Chap. 3). The purpose of this chapter on depression and the next (on anxiety) is to not just describe the studies that have found evidence for these mood issues, but to explore the parameters of these issues. For example, how severe is the depression? What is the cause?

Measurement of Depression

There are different ways of defining and measuring depression. In most PCOS research that assesses depression, measures of general depression are used; bipolar disorder (aka manic depression, discussed in the following chapter) and other specific types of depression (e.g. seasonal affective disorder) are not usually measured. In a clinical context, measurement of depression might involve ratings by a psychiatrist or psychologist, but in most psychological research, and most studies of PCOS, depression is measured by the participant's self-report on standardised questionnaires. One commonly used measure is the Beck's Depression Inventory (BDI; Beck et al. 1961) which consists of 21 items scored on a scale from 0 to 3. For example, in the first item, if the participant ticks the box indicating that they don't feel sad, this is scored as zero, and if they tick the box saying that they are so sad they can't stand it, this is scored at 3. Scores from the 21 items are added, and totals—which can range from 0 to 63—are used to identify six levels of depression. For example, according to BDI-II, scores below 14 indicate minimal depression (i.e. non-depressed), scores of 14 to 19 indicate 'mild depression', scores of 20 to 28 indicate moderate depression, and scores of 29 to 63 indicate severe depression. Both moderate and severe depression might be treated by a clinical psychologist, but only severe depression is generally considered 'clinical depression', or 'major depression' (Mayo Clinic 2019). Ultimately, the interpretation of questionnaire scores should be based on the clinical judgement of a psychologist (Beck et al. 1988) but in most research, patient self-report on questionnaires is used.

It's important to note that the scoring is very different when using the short version of a questionnaire. For example, in the short version of the BDI (the BDI Fast Screen, or BDI-FS), because there are fewer items, the threshold scores are lower: mild (5–8), moderate (9–12), and severe (>12). The same is true of other questionnaires, where different versions (different editions, different translations, versions for different age groups) may have different thresholds for scoring. This means that although comparing scores between groups (e.g. PCOS vs controls) in a study is usually fine, comparing actual scores across different studies requires attention to the specific scales being used. However, comparing the group differences (i.e. the effect size, whether *t*-value or Cohen's *d*, etc.) across studies can be done regardless of the measure being used, provided of course the measures are both valid and reliable measures of depression.

The BDI measures both depressed *state* (a feeling that might come or go depending on the situation) and depression *trait* (a feeling that endures across most situations), and does not differentiate between state and trait depression in the scoring. Some scales do make the distinction; for example, the State-Trait Depression Scales (Spielberger 1995) ask how the participant feels 'at this moment' on the 'state' scale, and how they 'generally' feel on the trait scale. This distinction can be useful in assessing how people's state depression scores lift in response to an intervention, which might not show up so clearly in measures that combine state and trait in a single score.

Role of PCOS-Related Issues in Depression

Although it is clear that depression is a risk in PCOS, attempts to identify the specific cause(s) of depression in PCOS have not provided a clear answer, probably because many variables could contribute to depression in PCOS (weight, acne, hirsutism, testosterone, etc.) both directly and indirectly (Barry et al. 2018). Day et al. (2018) suggest that depression in PCOS may have a genetic aspect related to BMI. However, genetic evidence should not be taken as a simple reductionist explanation, not least because other factors, both prenatal and postnatal, can modify the expression of genes. We should also be aware that on a basic human level, someone who is diagnosed with a condition that means their life will be impacted by a range of short- and long-term problems of varying degrees might well feel anxious and low in mood as a natural reaction.

Research suggests that although testosterone probably causes depression indirectly by causing the distressing symptoms of PCOS, the evidence for a direct effect of testosterone is weak (see Chaps. 4 and 7). In fact much of the evidence points to the symptoms, rather than testosterone levels, causing distress (Barry et al. 2011b, 2018; Pastore et al. 2011; Rahiminejad et al. 2014; Batool et al. 2016; Enjezab et al. 2017; Borghi et al. 2018).

In the section below the evidence that PCOS symptoms cause depression will be outlined.

Depression and Obesity in PCOS

In PCOS, obesity typically starts in adolescence and weight loss can be difficult. Bazarganipour et al. (2013) assessed 300 adult women with PCOS in Iran and found that higher BMI was associated with poorer body satisfaction. As well as the quality of life (QoL) impact of obesity (see Chap. 3), obese women tend to have lower self-esteem scores (Açmaz et al. 2013). Depression is often associated with obesity in PCOS (e.g. Cinar et al. 2011; Rasgon et al. 2003; Stapinska-Syniec et al. 2018) and in otherwise healthy women (Stunkard et al. 2003). There are exceptions, and some studies of PCOS and obesity have not found this relationship (McCook 2002; Hahn et al. 2005; Månsson et al. 2008) so we should be careful not to presume that all women with PCOS who are obese find their weight depressing, let alone are clinically depressed because of it.

The meta-analysis by Barry et al. (2011a) found that when obesity was accounted for, depression was reduced by a Hedge's g of 0.15, which is modest, given that a g of 0.2 is considered a 'small effect size'. Similarly, the meta-analysis by Cooney et al. (2017) found that when BMI was taken into account, the odds of women with PCOS being depressed was reduced from 4.18 times more than healthy women to 3.15 times more. This means that the increased prevalence of depressive symptoms in PCOS is not entirely independent of BMI, but BMI contributes a modest amount—an odds ratio (OR) of 1.03. As the authors of a seminal review of mental health in PCOS stated: 'obesity likely plays a part in the greater depression of women with PCOS, but it is clearly not the only contributor' (Himelein and Thatcher 2006, p. 724).

Several studies of PCOS have found that BMI and body weight are associated with increased depression (e.g. Milsom et al. 2013; Celik and Akbulut 2018b). It should not be surprising that weight impacts depression in PCOS, because not only might women have health and other concerns about being overweight, but also obesity worsens most of the symptoms of PCOS by causing an increase in insulin resistance (Celik and Akbulut 2018a). Although correlation does not prove causation, we can say that, in general, women who are overweight are more prone to depression, and about 80% of women with PCOS have an above-average BMI (Goyal and Dawood 2017). While it is true that sometimes people comfort eat for depression (Grucza et al. 2007), it is likely that the metabolic features of PCOS such as insulin resistance and lower metabolic rate (Farrell and Antoni 2010) contribute to weight gain which is difficult to lose, and common sense would suggest that this situation causes frustration and depression, or at least contributes to depression in PCOS.

It would be interesting to know whether women with the 'lean' variety of PCOS are less prone to depression. To date there have not been studies of adequate size to determine this with any accuracy, but Morotti et al. (2013) compared 33 normal-weight women with PCOS (BMI 19–25) to 22 healthy control women, and found BDI scores in both groups to be on the high side of normal (around 8 in both groups, with 9 as the threshold for mild depression on this version of the BDI). This lack of depression in a normal-weight PCOS group suggests that BMI is a factor in depression in PCOS, but a weakness of this study in understanding lean PCOS is that not all of the women in the PCOS group could be described as lean, as their BMIs were normal (in the UK today the normal range for women in women is 18.5–24.9). In any case, it seems possible that it is not quite so simple a task to compare lean women with PCOS to other women with PCOS women, as if this was a way to control for BMI in PCOS. This is because these two groups are probably unlike each other in ways other than just body weight: lean women with PCOS are probably more prone to disturbances in the hypothalamic-pituitary-adrenal (HPA) axis, and it is possible that hypothalamic dysfunction is implicated in the pathogenesis of lean PCOS (Goyal and Dawood 2017). Though more research is needed on the lean PCOS type, there is an argument for treating them as having a qualitatively different condition (or phenotype—see Chap. 1) compared to the 95% of other women with PCOS who are not lean.

Depression and Hirsutism in PCOS

Hirsutism is associated with elevated androgen levels in general, and varies with ethnicity (Young and Sinclair 1998). Kitzinger and Willmott (2002) interviewed 30 women with PCOS, and it emerged that PCOS is associated with feeling poorly adjusted to the feminine gender role, largely due to hirsutism and other effects of hyperandrogenism. Using the HADS, Lipton et al. (2006) found that 74% of 88 women who had problems with facial hair showed clinical levels of anxiety and 30% had clinical levels of depression. However, self-esteem (measured using the Rosenberg Self-Esteem Scales and The World Health Organization Quality of Life instrument, brief version (WHOQoL-BREF)) was not lower than normal in this group.

Elsenbruch et al. (2003) found that 50 women with PCOS felt particularly unattractive if hirsutism was a problem for them, and this caused them to experience sex as less satisfactory than 50 female controls. This was true even though the rate of sexual intercourse was similar in both groups, and also similar when BMI was taken into account. (See also the sections on 'sexual satisfaction' and 'body satisfaction' in Chap. 3).

Age, Depression, and BMI in PCOS

Depression in PCOS has seldom been measured longitudinally, though the evidence suggests that depression endures throughout the reproductive years of women with PCOS. One small study of women with PCOS (mean age 32 years old) suggested an increase in depression over roughly 1 to 2 years, mostly driven by concerns about weight (65% of the sample) and fertility (56.6% of the sample) (Kerchner et al. 2009).

In a study of 80 adolescents with PCOS and 50 age- and BMI-matched controls, Emeksiz et al. (2018) found higher depression in those with PCOS, and this depression was related to BMI. Milsom et al. (2013) found that depression was higher in 102 adolescents with PCOS presenting at a clinic compared to 1349 school-survey controls, but only when the PCOS girls had a higher BMI. Note that in this study the participants were recruited from different populations, which should make us slightly less certain about the validity of the findings.

Greenwood et al. (2019a) found that the rate of depression was relatively stable between around age 29 years old to around 34.5 years old, and was associated with BMI. Karjula et al. (2017) found, in a cohort of Finnish women, that the risk of depression in women with PCOS was higher than controls at age 31 and age 46. By far the longest of the longitudinal studies, another study by Greenwood et al. (2019b), assessed 83 women with PCOS who were aged 20–32 at baseline, and aged 45–57 at follow-up. They found that depression scores declined over the 25-year period in women with PCOS, and declined to a similar degree in 1044 control women. The difference in CES-D score was consistently around 2.5 points over the study period, but tended to be within the normal range (<16), that is, the mean scores did not indicate depression. An effect of ethnicity was seen, with black women with PCOS scoring highest (CES-D ~ 14), black women without PCOS and white women with PCOS scoring around 11, and white women without PCOS scoring around 8.

Whether depression endures in postmenopausal women with PCOS is a question that remains to be answered. It is possible that with the discomfort of menstrual and fertility issues behind them, and less pressure to be attractive, these women might be less depressed. On the other hand, the accumulated distress and disappointment of three decades with PCOS might leave some women disillusioned and more depressed, especially if PCOS has been a barrier to having a family. Research on depression in postmenopausal women with PCOS is a topic that needs further research.

Phenotype and Depression

An interesting question is whether PCOS phenotype has an impact on depression. This is an understudied question, especially regarding the lean phenotype. A study by Moran et al. (2012) found no effect on depression scores of National Institutes of Health (NIH)-diagnosed PCOS (hyperandrogenic) and women with a PCOS phenotype characterised by reproductive issues, but this study was perhaps too small to determine such effects. A similar study of around 100 Turkish women with PCOS with either the NIH phenotype or the non-NIH phenotype, and around 50 healthy female controls, found little difference in anxiety and depression scores by phenotype, though it found the expected difference between PCOS and controls (Cirik et al. 2016). Another study of Turkish women found no effect of phenotype on depression on the 226 participants with PCOS (Cinar et al. 2011). These findings support evidence that PCOS is linked to depression regardless of whether it is of the NIH phenotype or not (Day et al. 2018).

Cross-Cultural Findings Regarding Depression

Although PCOS affects similar rates of women across the world (Azziz 2006), we know that there are differences cross-culturally in the phenotypical expression of PCOS. For example, Zhao and Qiao (2013) found that East Asian women with PCOS have a high prevalence of metabolic syndrome, but lower BMI and a milder hyperandrogenic phenotype. We also know that concern about symptoms varies by culture; for example, Hashimoto et al. (2003) found that Brazilian women with PCOS were less concerned about being overweight than Austrian women with PCOS. But when it comes to cross-cultural differences in depression, it seems that there is not that much variation.

In a study of 272 women with PCOS and 295 controls using HADS, there was no difference in depression or anxiety scores in women with PCOS (Alur-Gupta et al. 2019). As expected, they found a higher prevalence of depressive symptoms in PCOS (26% vs 17%, $p < 0.01$) after adjusting for age, BMI, socioeconomic status, and race. This finding is supported by previous research from around the world. In the examples below, for the sake of comparability I have included studies that all used the same scale, either the HADS or the BDI. These two scales correlate well; for example, Cinar et al. (2011) found a correlation of $r = 0.72$. The meta-analysis by Dokras et al. (2011) shows (in their Table 2) a wide range of abnormal depression scores in PCOS (24–45%) compared to controls (2–22%). Comparing PCOS to controls on the BDI (none of the studies in Table 2 used the HADS), the rates in Italy were 24% versus 22% (Battaglia et al. 2008); in Greece 27% versus 9% (Laggari et al. 2009); in the US 24% versus 22% (Himelein and Thatcher 2006); in Turkey 33% versus 12% (Adali et al. 2008); again in Turkey 35% versus 17% (Soyupek et al. 2008); and in Germany 45% versus 16% (Benson et al. 2008). Since the time of publication of that meta-analysis in 2011, other studies have reported similar findings. For example, using the BDI with 73 women with PCOS and 116 healthy control women in Iran, Salehifar et al. (2016) found rates of severe depression in 21% of PCOS patients and 8% of controls. Zehra et al. (2015) assessed 225 women with PCOS and 200 healthy controls in Pakistan, and using the cut-off of a HADS score of 8 (mild depression), they found higher rates of depression in PCOS (31%) than controls (6%). Overall these studies show that across most of the world, around a quarter to a third of women with PCOS indicate signs of depression compared to about a fifth of healthy women. However, although the evidence doesn't show a strong pattern of variation in depression scores across cultures, absence of evidence is not evidence of absence; more studies, and larger studies, are needed in more parts of the world, especially Asia and Southern Africa.

Although it is in some ways difficult to identify rates of depression exactly (for the reasons cited in the section on methodology below), the evidence to date suggests that rates of depression are fairly similar in women with PCOS cross-culturally. The slightly greater variation in differences in levels of depression within each of the two groups separately (PCOS and controls in each country) can probably be explained to some degree by normal sampling variation; for example, if you conducted ten studies of women with PCOS in London, with 100 women in each of the studies, you would most likely observe slightly different rates of depression in each of the studies. In the same way, the small differences (a quarter to a third rate of depression in PCOS) probably don't reflect large cultural differences, although it is likely that culture will have some impact, for example, in regard to fertility problems, because some cultures value fertility above other issues impacted by PCOS.

Genetics and Depression in PCOS

A fascinating study of 12,628 Swedish female twins born from 1959 to 1985 found that women with PCOS had double the risk of major depression in their lifetime (Cesta et al. 2017). They also found that they had greater tendencies to neuroticism, and that the three variables—PCOS, depression, and neuroticism—shared a common genetic link. (Neuroticism is discussed in more detail in Chap. 3.)

Inflammation and Depression in PCOS

It's long been known that depression can be correlated with proinflammatory cytokines (Anisman et al. 1999), and some anti-depressants reduce proinflammatory cytokine production (Kenis and Maes 2002). Chronic stress and depression can impact the immune system causing increased immune activity, thus increasing the risk of diabetes, cardiovascular disease (CVD), and cancer (Raison et al. 2006). Although we can't say for certain that this correlation implies causation, the weight of evidence appears to point in that direction.

Farrell and Antoni (2010) suggest that chronically elevated inflammatory markers may be the cause of fatigue, depressed mood, social withdrawal, and sleep disturbance in PCOS. They suggest that cytokines weaken the blood-brain barrier, causing serotonin deficiency and chronic elevation of stress hormones. This is an interesting hypothesis that deserves further research.

How Severe Is Depression in PCOS?

It is possible that the severity of depression is overestimated due to the use of clinical samples in PCOS research; clinical samples involve women with symptoms severe enough for medical attention, and the experiences of these women might not reflect the experiences of women with PCOS who have less severe symptoms, and perhaps are even undiagnosed (Azziz et al. 2016).

The severity of depression in PCOS is an important issue. Knowing the levels of severity and the rates of these levels helps us to prepare the appropriate interventions. Unrealistically high estimates might prepare us to deliver services that are less appropriate for those with lower levels of depression. An accurate assessment is important, and requires that we have a clear understanding of the available evidence.

The meta-analysis by Barry et al. (2011a) found that, based on the most commonly used measure of depression (the BDI), although the difference between depression in women with PCOS and controls was of statistical significance (Hedges' $g = 0.60$, $p < 0.00001$), the difference in mean scores (11.47 vs 7.31) indicates, on average, mild depression in the PCOS groups and no depression in the control groups.

Similarly, a meta-analysis by Cooney et al. (2017) reported that 'depressive symptoms' are around twice as common in PCOS than other women: 36.6% versus 14.2% and that moderate to severe depression is around four times more common in PCOS. Their Supplementary Table III shows that of the 30 studies cited in their meta-analysis, 23 reported depression rates and 9 identified the specific level of depression (mild, moderate or severe). Based on this subset of 9 studies, the mean rates of mild depression were PCOS = 23.4%, controls = 15.0%; of moderate depression were PCOS = 19.3%, controls = 5.6%; and of severe depression were PCOS = 5.7%, controls = 0.9%. This breakdown of information is important in showing that severe depression is six times more likely in PCOS compared to controls, and moderate depression is almost four times more likely. We could also note that around one in five women had moderate depression, and one in twenty had severe depression.

The meta-analyses by Barry et al. (2011a) and Cooney et al. (2017) highlight two important issues about reporting the severity of depression: firstly, reporting only the group mean rather than rates, which is done by Barry et al. (2011a) and about a third of the other studies in this field, can create a 'one-size-fits-all' view of the degree of depression, which will not represent the findings with sufficient nuance. Although interval/ratio data is more flexible than categorical data and can be used in a wider variety of complex linear statistical tests, for the purposes of reporting clinical data, by itself the group mean lacks sufficient information. Secondly, in order that readers can clearly understand how depressed the groups are, the specific degree of depression, according to cut-offs for the specific scale, should be reported clearly in the main text of the paper, if not the abstract, rather than supplementary tables, as done by (Cooney et al. 2017).

The importance of clarity in the presentation of research data is that clinical services can best be prepared to meet the needs of patients when based on clear information of clinical relevance. Not everybody has access to the full text of research papers, so it is important to be clear about the rate and severity in the abstract. For example, saying in the abstract that 67–71% of women with PCOS 'were classified as depressed', and clarifying three pages later that most of these women were at most minimally depressed, and only around 14% were severely depressed, is not a way of reporting that 'refines our understanding of depression' in PCOS (Barnard et al. 2007, p. 2279). The confusion is caused by reporting the rate of depression using the minimum cut-off without saying that this figure includes clinical and non-clinical depression scores, and is not uncommon in PCOS research (e.g. seen in Cirik et al. 2016). Greater precision should be used in reporting rates of depression, as with any other potentially serious clinical condition, in order that confusion can be avoided and appropriate services provided (Barry et al. 2014).

Clinical Versus Community Samples

One relatively large and well-controlled study put the estimate of clinical depression in women with PCOS at almost 30% (using the BDI) compared to 5% for controls (Cinar et al. 2011). In this study, there were 226 PCOS patients and 85 BMI-matched healthy controls, and validated measures of depression (the HADS and BDI) were used. Although this would appear to be a robust study, we should remember that the sample was from endocrinology clinics; in other words, the women in this study were troubled enough by their symptoms that they sought medical help. If we compare this to an online sample (e.g. Barnard et al. 2007) which is likely to include women who have PCOS with symptoms not severe enough to be at an endocrinology clinic, we find that only around half that number report being severely depressed.

Are Women with PCOS More Suicidal than Other Women?

The findings of some studies paint a bleak picture of mental health in PCOS. For example, in a very widely cited Swedish study, Månsson et al. (2008) reported in their abstract that suicide attempts were seven times more common in PCOS than in age-matched healthy control women. This is an alarmingly difference. The results section of the paper reveals that 14% (7 of 49 women) of the women with PCOS had attempted suicide, compared to 2% of controls (one of 49 women). So what might have caused such high rates of suicide attempts in Månsson et al. (2008)? There are several possible interpretations. Firstly, we could take the finding at face value and accept that women with PCOS are seven times more likely than other women to try to kill themselves. However, there are alternative explanations. Most obviously, the sample size was relatively small, and the finding of suicide attempts might be due to chance rather than being representative of that average woman with PCOS. In general, studies with larger sample sizes yield findings that are more representative of the overall population that they are supposed to represent. (In this particular case the 'population' is 'women with PCOS'.)

Secondly, we don't know how serious or how recent these suicide attempts were. Månsson et al. (2008) modified the MINI International Neuropsychiatric Interview (Sheehan et al. 1998), leaving out questions on the severity of the attempt, and asked just one question about whether a suicide attempt had ever been made rather than whether an attempt had been made in the past month (Ayhan et al. 2017). These adaptations, although perhaps justifiable for pilot research, mean that Månsson's findings can't be compared to other studies using the MINI. More importantly, we should note that people are far more likely to report a suicide attempt in their lifetime rather than in the past month, and are more likely to make a non-serious attempt than one requiring hospitalisation (Roaldset et al. 2012). In other words, like the problem with specifying the severity of depression discussed above, the definition of suicide attempt is such that the least serious attempts are counted as much as the most serious.

Thirdly, there is the issue of how well controlled the variables were in the study. Although Månsson et al. (2008) controlled very well for age, the PCOS group reported higher rates of sickness benefits than controls (24% vs 8%) and a smaller number of children (45% vs 61%). It has long been known that better health and having a family are protective against suicidality (Durkheim 1897, 2005), but it is difficult to successfully control for these variables in studies of PCOS, because they are likely to be systematically different in PCOS and healthy women. The same problem applies to controlling for BMI (see 'Methodological Issues' section below), which was 29.1 in the PCOS group and 23.5 in the controls in the Månsson et al. (2008) sample. It would have been interesting to see an analysis of how much suicide attempts were related to sickness, fertility, or BMI, despite the inevitable difficulties of being truly able to control for these variables in PCOS research.

So are women with PCOS more suicidal than other women? There are not many studies of suicide risk in PCOS and undoubtedly more good quality research is needed on this important issue. Using the BDI, Hollinrake et al. (2007) found 12% of depressed women with PCOS had suicidal thoughts but did not report the rate of suicidal thoughts in the control group, despite actually having a control group. Control groups are useful, provided they are similar to the PCOS in group in other ways relevant to the study (e.g. age, BMI, and—with reference to Månsson et al.—health and family size). For example, although Hollinrake found

12% suicidal *thoughts* in depressed women with PCOS, this—unlike suicide *attempts*—is not particularly unusual in women in the general population, and varies by country, for example, 8.8% in Finland and 16.5% in Ireland (Casey et al. 2006).

Scaruffi et al. (2014) found, using the Rorschach test, 8.1% at risk for suicide in women with PCOS compared to 6% of healthy control women. This group difference (8.1% vs 6%) is much smaller than the Månsson et al. (2008) finding of a seven-fold difference (14% versus 2%). But perhaps the best evidence to date on this topic is an epidemiological study from Sweden (Cesta et al. 2016), the same country studied by Månsson et al., which found that the risk of attempted suicide in women with PCOS was much less pronounced. Their study of 24,385 women with PCOS and 243,850 without PCOS found that the risk of attempted suicide was 3.4% vs 2.4%. In relative terms, the risk was 41% higher in women with PCOS than for other women (OR = 1.41). Once the presence of psychiatric disorders was adjusted for, there was no significant difference between women with PCOS and other women (adjusted OR 1.05). Nor was there a difference in the risk of completed suicides (adjusted OR = 0.86).

Methodological Issues in PCOS Research

Study Design and Sample Size

Research into the psychological aspects of PCOS is relatively new having started in the mid-1990s, and the preponderance of relatively small cross-sectional studies in this field reflects the early exploratory efforts of researchers. The small study sizes probably also reflect the lack of funding for this topic; large studies can be expensive, and PCOS is not generally considered as high a priority for the major funding bodies as conditions such as cancer or diabetes, despite the fact that PCOS carries the risk for both. Although in PCOS research there are some larger studies and some longitudinal studies, more large studies are needed in order that we can gather better evidence to more clearly understand this complex condition. Large sample sizes ($N > 200$) are preferable, as they give a better chance of generalisable findings that are more representative of the PCOS population (provided that sampling is not biased), and give more statistical power and allow for more sophisticated statistical tests (e.g. multiple linear regression). Studies should always be large enough to sufficiently power statistical tests, and preferably based on appropriate calculations (Tabachnick and Fidell 2006).

Free software is available for this purpose, for example, G*Power (Faul et al. 2009). Longitudinal studies—ones that follow women's progress over a course of time—are preferable to cross-sectional studies which assess women only at one point in time. This is because longitudinal studies can identify the development of a condition over time, and also allow the identification of the variables that cause changes in health over that time. Other designs are preferred to cross-sectional studies too, especially randomised controlled trials (RCTs) in which variables can be tightly controlled, and the effect of specific variables seen from one time point to another.

Cut-Offs

There can be a tendency to all-or-nothing thinking when it comes to research into depression in PCOS. For example, the tendency to use the lowest threshold for depression as a marker for depression per se shows a lack of subtlety of interpretation of psychometric scales. Sometimes cut-offs can be confusing, and can be at different points for different versions of the same scale. A classic error is of accidentally overlapping categories; for example, in Table 2 of Radhakrishnan and Verghese (2018) HADS scores of 8–11 were identified as borderline, and 11–21 were abnormal, which puts women who scored '11' into two categories. The authors had stated correctly in the method section of their paper that a score of 8–10 is mild, and 11–21 is abnormal, which shows how easy it is to accidentally overlap the categories.

Type 2 Error for Small Effects

Similarly, the notion that a consistently small effect is an irrelevant effect lacks nuance. For example, the link between BMI and depression is small (e.g. the Hedge's g of 0.15 found by Barry et al. [2011a] is technically not quite big enough to be called a small effect), but this trend appears consistently enough to be of interest to us. It might be the kind of effect that is not quite statistically significant, but might be clinically significant in terms of the impact on the patient's experience. So although BMI does not completely account for depression in PCOS, it probably contributes to it. PCOS is a complex condition and inevitably explanations regarding the cause of psychological issues are going to be subtle and multifactorial.

Controlling the Uncontrollable

Perhaps the major methodological issue, and one that is impossible to fully resolve, is trying to control for the impact of BMI in studies of PCOS (e.g. Cirik et al. 2016), through either matching participants or statistical methods (analysis of covariance, or ANCOVA). The problem is that when two groups systematically differ on a variable, which is the case when most women with PCOS have a higher BMI than most healthy women, then that variable simply cannot be realistically controlled for. The effect of trying to do so is to reduce differences between the PCOS and the control group (e.g. Elsenbruch et al. 2003). Typically, matching or using ANCOVA in this situation may cause a type 2 error, that is, the error of overlooking a significant finding. (For an excellent discussion of this issue, see Miller and Chapman 2001). Because there is no real solution to this problem, the best thing to do is to try different methods of controlling the variable, such as matching with different types of control group (e.g. subfertile non-PCOS control group, a PCOS-lean control group, a non-PCOS hirsute control group), and noting how the findings change according to the different groups, thereby gaining insights into different facets of the relationship.

With the above caveat in mind, studies that control for BMI often find that women with PCOS still have significantly higher depression than normative samples (Keegan et al. 2003) and age-/weight-matched controls (Weiner et al. 2004), suggesting that BMI is not the only variable that is causing depression in PCOS. For example, Hollinrake et al. (2007) found that a subgroup of obese women with PCOS ($n = 73$) were significantly more at risk of clinical depression than obese controls. This might indicate that the other symptoms of PCOS added to the depression risk, but it could also be that the type of obesity seen in PCOS is more distressing, because android (or central) obesity has a less feminine appearance than gynoid obesity (where weight gain is on the hips) and is more resistant to ordinary dieting (Marsh and Brand-Miller 2005). There is evidence that in general, central obesity ('apple shaped' body rather than 'pear shaped') is considered less attractive in women in many cultures (Brown 1991). This body shape is caused by elevated androgens and is typical of PCOS. This cross-cultural evidence suggests that although it maybe be secondary in QoL terms to other issues, elevated BMI is likely to impact the wellbeing of women with PCOS regardless of their cultural background. A difficulty of android obesity is that it contributes, in a vicious cycle, to higher androgen levels via the decrease in aromatase activity in adipose tissue (Wake et al. 2007) so we should expect that BMI has a global impact on features affected by testosterone.

BMI Versus WHR

A related measurement issue in PCOS is that although BMI is typically measured as an index of obesity, it is likely that the waist-to-hip ratio (WHR) is a better measure of android or central obesity than BMI (Carranza-Lira et al. 2006). BMI might not be an accurate measure of health status, because women with PCOS have more lean muscle mass than healthy women, which is surprising (Carmina et al. 2009), because muscle tissue typically helps to burn calories, yet women with PCOS tend to have a lower basal metabolic rate than do healthy women of a similar age and BMI (Georgopoulos et al. 2009).

Overall, the evidence suggests that obesity contributes to depression in PCOS, but one or more other factors are also contributors.

Main Recommendations Regarding Research in PCOS

Reporting the Levels of Depression

When measuring psychological factors, have a psychologist (preferably a health psychologist) on your research team, and one who is experienced in the administration of psychometric tests. The rates of depression and group means (±SD) should be reported. The degree of depression should be made clear at every point in the published research paper; for example, say '30% of women had depression scores indicating mild depression; 20% had scores indicating moderate depression; 5% had scores indicating severe depression; 45% of scores indicated no depression'. Rates of categories of depression should not be combined, especially in the abstract (e.g. 'moderate or severe depression'). Mean ± SD scores can also be reported (if parametric assumptions are met), and the degree of depression the means represent. For example, 'The mean ± SD scores shown in Table X indicate mild depression in the PCOS group and no depression in the control group'. If parametric assumptions are not met, then group medians and ranges can be reported.

Make sure the paper is written in a way that is sensitive to these nuances. Some readers will have access to only the abstract, so it is especially important that the abstract doesn't contain 'dramatic' information that later in the paper is revealed to be less dramatic. The intention might be to draw attention in the abstract to an important issue, but the effect might be to leave the reader with the wrong impression of the findings. It might be important to make clear to the journal editor that this kind of information should, for ethical reasons, be stated in the abstract.

Other Methodological Issues

Be sure that the study's statistician is aware of problems of controlling for BMI in PCOS research, because these may influence the research design. Structural equation modelling should be considered as a way to understand the complex interrelation between the many variables implicated in depression in PCOS.

As a general rule always use validated measures, and if possible use short versions because these are more user-friendly, especially if a battery of questionnaires are being administered.

Sometimes statistically significant findings are not of clinical significance, for example, if the scores of both groups are within the same category of depression.

In summary, good research on the causes of depression in PCOS will lead to the best possible treatment options, so good quality research by expert research teams is important. PCOS is an incredibly complex syndrome and relatively difficult to research. Learning to adapt our research methods to meet the challenges of PCOS is a difficult process, but one that will help this important new field to make the breakthrough findings that will benefit everyone.

References

Açmaz, G., Albayrak, E., Acmaz, B., Başer, M., Soyak, M., Zararsız, G., & İpekMüderris, İ. (2013). Level of anxiety, depression, self-esteem, social anxiety, and quality of life among the women with polycystic ovary syndrome. *The Scientific World Journal, 2013*, 7.

Adali, E., Yildizhan, R., Kurdoglu, M., Kolusari, A., Edirne, T., Sahin, H. G., … Kamaci, M. (2008). The relationship between clinico-biochemical characteristics and psychiatric distress in young women with polycystic ovary syndrome. *Journal of International Medical Research, 36*(6), 1188–1196.

Alur-Gupta, S., Lee, I., Chemerinski, A., Chang, L., & Dokras, A. (2019, March 25). Racial differences in anxiety, depression, and quality of life between white and black women with PCOS and controls. *Endo2019 conference*. Session OR25—OR25. Reproductive endocrinology in the female: Lessons from human and mouse models. Retrieved from https://www.abstractsonline.com/pp8/#!/5752/presentation/17064.

Anisman, H., Ravindran, A. V., Griffiths, J., & Merali, Z. (1999). Endocrine and cytokine correlates of major depression and dysthymia with typical or atypical features. *Molecular Psychiatry, 4*, 182–188.

Ayhan, G., Arnal, R., Basurko, C., Pastre, A., Pinganaud, E., Sins, D., … Nacher, M. (2017). Suicide risk among prisoners in French Guiana: Prevalence and predictive factors. *BMC Psychiatry, 17*(1), 156.

Azziz, R. (2006). Controversy in clinical endocrinology: Diagnosis of polycystic ovarian syndrome: The Rotterdam criteria are premature. *The Journal of Clinical Endocrinology and Metabolism, 9*, 781–785.

Azziz, R., Carmina, E., Chen, Z., Dunaif, A., Laven, J. S., Legro, R. S., … Yildiz, B. O. (2016). Polycystic ovary syndrome. *Nature Reviews. Disease Primers, 2*, 16057.

Barnard, L., Ferriday, D., Guenther, N., Strauss, B., Balen, A. H., & Dye, L. (2007). Quality of life and psychological well being in polycystic ovary syndrome. *Human Reproduction, 22*, 2279–2286.

Barry, J. A., Hardiman, P. J., Saxby, B. K., & Kuczmierczyk, A. (2011a). Testosterone and mood dysfunction in women with polycystic ovarian syndrome compared to subfertile controls. *Journal of Psychosomatic Obstetrics and Gynecology, 32*(2), 104–111.

Barry, J. A., Hardiman, P. J., Saxby, B. K., & Kuczmierczyk, A. (2011b). Testosterone and mood dysfunction in women with polycystic ovarian syndrome compared to subfertile controls. *Journal of Psychosomatic Obstetrics and Gynecology, 32*, 104–111.

Barry, J. A., Kuczmierczyk, A. R., & Hardiman, P. J. (2014). Reporting the rates of depression in polycystic ovary syndrome (PCOS). *The Journal of Sexual Medicine, 11*(7), 1882–1883.

Barry, J. A., Leite, N., Sivarajah, N., Keevil, B., Owen, L., Miranda, L. C., … Hardiman, P. (2017). Relaxation and guided imagery significantly reduces androgen levels and distress in Polycystic Ovary Syndrome: Pilot study. *Contemporary Hypnosis and Integrative Therapy, 32*(1), 21–29.

Barry, J. A., Qu, F., & Hardiman, P. J. (2018). An exploration of the hypothesis that testosterone is implicated in the psychological functioning of women with polycystic ovary syndrome (PCOS). *Medical Hypotheses, 110*, 42–45.

Batool, S., ul ain Ahmed, F., Ambreen, A., Sheikh, A., & Faryad, N. (2016). Depression and anxiety in women with polycystic ovary syndrome and its biochemical associates. *Journal of South Asian Federation of Obstetrics and Gynaecology, 8*(1), 44–47.

Battaglia, C., Nappi, R. E., Mancini, F., Cianciosi, A., Persico, N., Busacchi, P., … Sisti, G. (2008). PCOS, sexuality, and clitoral vascularisation: A pilot study. *The Journal of Sexual Medicine, 5*, 2886–2894.

Bazarganipour, F., Ziaei, S., Montazeri, A., Foroozanfard, F., Kazemnejad, A., & Faghihzadeh, S. (2013). Body image satisfaction and self-esteem status among the patients with polycystic ovary syndrome. *Iranian Journal of Reproductive Medicine, 11*(10), 829.

Bazarganipour, F., Ziaei, S., Montazeri, A., Foroozanfard, F., Kazemnejad, A., & Faghihzadeh, S. (2014). Health-related quality of life in patients with polycystic ovary syndrome (PCOS): A model-based study of predictive factors. *The Journal of Sexual Medicine, 11*, 1023–1032.

Beck, A. T., Ward, C. H., Mendelson, M., Mock, J., & Erbaugh, J. (1961). An inventory for measuring depression. *Archives of General Psychiatry, 4*, 561–571.

Beck, A. T., Steer, R. A., & Garbin, M. G. (1988). Psychometric properties of the Beck Depression Inventory: Twenty-five years of evaluation. *Clinical Psychology Review, 8*, 77–100.

Benson, S., Janssen, O. E., Hahn, S., Tan, S., Dietz, T., Mann, K., … Elsenbruch, S. (2008). Obesity, depression, and chronic low-grade inflammation in women with polycystic ovary syndrome. *Brain, Behavior, and Immunity, 22*(2), 177–184.

Borghi, L., Leone, D., Vegni, E., Galiano, V., Lepadatu, C., Sulpizio, P., & Garzia, E. (2018). Psychological distress, anger and quality of life in polycystic ovary syndrome: Associations with biochemical, phenotypical and socio-demographic factors. *Journal of Psychosomatic Obstetrics and Gynecology, 39*(2), 128–137.

Brown, P. J. (1991). Culture and the evolution of obesity. *Human Nature, 2*, 31–57.

Carmina, E., Guastella, E., Longo, R. A., Rini, G. B., & Lobo, R. A. (2009). Correlates of increased lean muscle mass in women with polycystic ovary syndrome. *European Journal of Endocrinology, 161*(4), 583–589.

Carranza-Lira, S., Velasco Díaz, G., Olivares, A., Chán Verdugo, R., & Herrera, J. (2006). Correlation of Kupperman's index with estrogen and androgen levels, according to weight and body fat distribution in postmenopausal women from Mexico City. *International Journal of Fertility and Women's Medicine, 51*, 83–88.

Casey, P. R., Dunn, G., Kelly, B. D., Birkbeck, G., Dalgard, O. S., Lehtinen, V., … ODIN Group. (2006). Factors associated with suicidal ideation in the general population: Five-centre analysis from the ODIN study. *The British Journal of Psychiatry, 189*(5), 410–415.

Celik, E., & Akbulut, G. (2018a). The relationship between obesity and insulin resistance in polycystic ovary syndrome. *Clinical Nutrition, 37*, S145.

Celik, E., & Akbulut, G. (2018b). The relationship between obesity and depression in polycystic ovary syndrome. *Clinical Nutrition, 37*, S145.

Cesta, C. E., Mansson, M., Palm, C., Lichtenstein, P., Iliadou, A. N., & Landen, M. (2016). Polycystic ovary syndrome and psychiatric disorders: Co-morbidity and heritability in a nationwide Swedish cohort. *Psychoneuroendocrinology, 73*, 196–203.

Cesta, C. E., Kuja-Halkola, R., Lehto, K., Iliadou, A. N., & Landén, M. (2017). Polycystic ovary syndrome, personality, and depression: A twin study. *Psychoneuroendocrinology, 85*, 63–68.

Cinar, N., Kizilarslanoglu, M. C., Harmanci, A., Aksoy, D. Y., Bozdag, G., Demir, B., & Yildiz, B. O. (2011). Depression, anxiety and cardiometabolic risk in polycystic ovary syndrome. *Human Reproduction, 26*(12), 3339–3345.

Cirik, D. A., Dilbaz, B., Aksakal, S. E., Kotan, Z., Özelçi, R., Akpinar, F., & Mollamahmutoğlu, L. (2016). Do anxiety and depression statuses differ in different polycystic ovary syndrome phenotypes? *Turkish Journal of Medical Sciences, 46*(6), 1846–1853.

Cooney, L. G., Lee, I., Sammel, M. D., & Dokras, A. (2017). High prevalence of moderate and severe depressive and anxiety symptoms in polycystic ovary syndrome: A systematic review and meta-analysis. *Human Reproduction, 32*(5), 1075–1091.

Day, F., Karaderi, T., Jones, M. R., Meun, C., He, C., Drong, A., ... Magi, R. (2018). Large-scale genome-wide meta-analysis of polycystic ovary syndrome suggests shared genetic architecture for different diagnosis criteria. *PLoS Genetics, 14*(12), e1007813.

Dokras, A., Clifton, S., Futterweit, W., & Wild, R. (2011). Increased risk for abnormal depression scores in women with polycystic ovary syndrome: A systematic review and meta-analysis. *Obstetrics and Gynecology, 117*, 145–152.

Durkheim, E. (2005). *Suicide: A study in sociology*. London: Routledge.

Elsenbruch, S., Hahn, S., Kowalsky, D., Offner, A. H., Schedlowski, M., Mann, K., & Janssen, O. E. (2003). Quality of life, psychosocial well-being, and sexual satisfaction in women with polycystic ovary syndrome. *The Journal of Clinical Endocrinology and Metabolism, 88*, 5801–5807.

Emeksiz, H. C., Bideci, A., Nalbantoğlu, B., Nalbantoğlu, A., Celik, C., Yulaf, Y., ... Cinaz, P. (2018). Anxiety and depression states of adolescents with polycystic ovary syndrome. *Turkish Journal of Medical Sciences, 48*(3), 531–536.

Enjezab, B., Eftekhar, M., & Ghadiri-Anari, A. (2017). Association between severity of depression and clinico-biochemical markers of polycystic ovary syndrome. *Electronic Physician, 9*(11), 5820.

Farrell, K., & Antoni, M. H. (2010). Insulin resistance, obesity, inflammation, and depression in polycystic ovary syndrome: Biobehavioral mechanisms and interventions. *Fertility and Sterility, 94*(5), 1565–1574.

Faul, F., Erdfelder, E., Buchner, A., & Lang, A. G. (2009). Statistical power analyses using G∗ Power 3.1: Tests for correlation and regression analyses. *Behavior Research Methods, 41*(4), 1149–1160.

Georgopoulos, N. A., Saltamavros, A. D., Vervita, V., Karkoulias, K., Adonakis, G., Decavalas, G., ... Kyriazopoulou, V. (2009). Basal metabolic rate is decreased in women with polycystic ovary syndrome and biochemical hyperandrogenemia and is associated with insulin resistance. *Fertility and Sterility, 92*(1), 250–255.

Goyal, M., & Dawood, A. S. (2017). Debates regarding lean patients with polycystic ovary syndrome: A narrative review. *Journal of Human Reproductive Sciences, 10*(3), 154.

Greenwood, E. A., Pasch, L. A., Shinkai, K., Cedars, M. I., & Huddleston, H. G. (2015). Putative role for insulin resistance in depression risk in polycystic ovary syndrome. *Fertility and Sterility, 104*(3), 707–714.

Greenwood, E. A., Pasch, L. A., Cedars, M. I., Legro, R. S., Huddleston, H. G., & Network, H. D. R. M., & Eunice Kennedy Shriver National Institute of Child Health. (2018). Association among depression, symptom experience, and quality of life in polycystic ovary syndrome. *American Journal of Obstetrics and Gynecology, 219*(3), 279–2e1.

Greenwood, E. A., Pasch, L. A., Shinkai, K., Cedars, M. I., & Huddleston, H. G. (2019a). Clinical course of depression symptoms and predictors of enduring depression risk in women with polycystic ovary syndrome: Results of a longitudinal study. *Fertility and Sterility, 111*(1), 147–156.

Greenwood, E. A., Yaffe, K., Wellons, M. F., Cedars, M. I., & Huddleston, H. G. (2019b). Depression over the lifespan in a population-based cohort of women with polycystic ovary syndrome: Longitudinal analysis. *The Journal of Clinical Endocrinology & Metabolism, 104*(7), 2809–2819.

Grucza, R. A., Przybeck, T. R., & Cloninger, C. R. (2007). Prevalence and correlates of binge eating disorder in a community sample. *Comprehensive Psychiatry, 48*, 124–131.

Hahn, S., Janssen, O. E., Tan, S., Pleger, K., Mann, K., Schedlowski, M., … Elsenbruch, S. (2005). Clinical and psychological correlates of quality-of-life in polycystic ovary syndrome. *European Journal of Endocrinology, 153*(6), 853–860.

Hashimoto, D. M., Schmid, J., Martins, F. M., Fonseca, A. M., Andrade, L. H. B., Kirchengast, S., & Eggers, S. (2003). The impact of the weight status on subjective symptomatology of the polycystic ovary syndrome: A cross-cultural comparison between Brazilian and Austrian women. *Anthropologischer Anzeiger, 61*(3), 297–310.

Himelein, M. J., & Thatcher, S. S. (2006). Depression and body image among women with polycystic ovary syndrome. *Journal of Health Psychology, 11*, 613–625.

Hollinrake, E., Abreu, A., Maifeld, M., Van Voorhis, B. J., & Dokras, A. (2007). Increased risk of depressive disorders in women with polycystic ovary syndrome. *Fertility and Sterility, 87*, 1369–1376.

Karjula, S., Morin-Papunen, L., Auvinen, J., Ruokonen, A., Puukka, K., Franks, S., … Piltonen, T. T. (2017). Psychological distress is more prevalent in fertile age and premenopausal women with PCOS symptoms—15-year follow-up. *The Journal of Clinical Endocrinology & Metabolism, 102*, 1861–1869.

Keegan, A., Liao, L. M., & Boyle, M. (2003). 'Hirsutism': A psychological analysis. *Journal of Health Psychology, 8*, 327–345.

Kenis, G., & Maes, M. (2002). Effects of antidepressants on the production of cytokines. *The International Journal of Neuropsychopharmacology, 5*, 401–412.

Kerchner, A., Lester, W., Stuart, S. P., & Dokras, A. (2009). Risk of depression and other mental health disorders in women with polycystic ovary syndrome: A longitudinal study. *Fertility and Sterility, 91*(1), 207–212.

Kitzinger, C., & Willmott, J. (2002). 'The thief of womanhood': Women's experience of polycystic ovarian syndrome. *Social Science & Medicine, 54*, 349–361.

Laggari, V., Diareme, S., Christogiorgos, S., Deligeoroglou, E., Christopoulos, P., Tsiantis, J., & Creatsas, G. (2009). Anxiety and depression in adolescents with polycystic ovary syndrome and Mayer-Rokitansky-Küster-Hauser syndrome. *Journal of Psychosomatic Obstetrics and Gynecology, 30*(2), 83–88.

Lipton, M. G., Sherr, L., Elford, J., Rustin, M. H., & Clayton, W. J. (2006). Women living with facial hair: The psychological and behavioral burden. *Journal of Psychosomatic Research, 61*, 161–168.

Månsson, M., Holte, J., Landin-Wilhelmsen, K., Dahlgren, E., Johansson, A., & Landén, M. (2008). Women with polycystic ovary syndrome are often depressed or anxious—A case control study. *Psychoneuroendocrinology, 33*(8), 1132–1138.

Marsh, K., & Brand-Miller, J. (2005). The optimal diet for women with polycystic ovary syndrome? *British Journal of Nutrition, 94*, 154–165.

Mayo Clinic. (2019). *What is clinical depression?* Retrieved May 28, 2019, from https://www.mayoclinic.org/diseases-conditions/depression/expert-answers/clinical-depression/faq-20057770.

McCook, J. G. (2002). *The influence of hyperandrogenism, obesity and infertility on the psychosocial health and wellbeing of women with polycystic ovary syndrome.* Unpublished doctoral dissertation, University of Michigan.

Miller, G. A., & Chapman, J. P. (2001). Misunderstanding analysis of covariance. *Journal of Abnormal Psychology, 110*(1), 40.

Milsom, S. R., Nair, S. M., Ogilvie, C. M., Stewart, J. M., & Merry, S. N. (2013). Polycystic ovary syndrome and depression in New Zealand adolescents. *Journal of Pediatric and Adolescent Gynecology, 26*(3), 142–147.

Monzani, F., Pucci, F., Caraccio, N., Bagnolesi, A., Molli, D., Fenu, A., & Prunetti, C. (1994). Psychological and psychopathological correlates in the polycystic ovary syndrome (PCOS). *Medicina–Psicosomatica, 39*, 225–236.

Moran, L. J., Deeks, A. A., Gibson-Helm, M. E., & Teede, H. J. (2012). Psychological parameters in the reproductive phenotypes of polycystic ovary syndrome. *Human Reproduction, 27*, 2082–2088.

Morotti, E., Persico, N., Battaglia, B., Fabbri, R., Meriggiola, M. C., Venturoli, S., & Battaglia, C. (2013). Body imaging and sexual behavior in lean women with polycystic ovary syndrome. *The Journal of Sexual Medicine, 10*, 2752–2760.

Pastore, L. M., Patrie, J. T., Morris, W. L., Dalal, P., & Bray, M. J. (2011). Depression symptoms and body dissatisfaction association among polycystic ovary syndrome women. *Journal of Psychosomatic Research, 71*(4), 270–276.

Radhakrishnan, R., & Verghese, A. (2018). A study on anxiety and depression among patients with polycystic ovary syndrome. *Journal of Drug Delivery and Therapeutics, 8*(5-s), 338–340.

Rahiminejad, M. E., Moaddab, A., Rabiee, S., Esna-Ashari, F., Borzouei, S., & Hosseini, S. M. (2014). The relationship between clinicobiochemical markers and depression in women with polycystic ovary syndrome. *Iranian Journal of Reproductive Medicine, 12*(12), 811.

Raison, C. L., Capuron, L., & Miller, A. H. (2006). Cytokines sing the blues: Inflammation and the pathogenesis of depression. *Trends in Immunology, 27*, 24–31.

Rasgon, N. L., Rao, R. C., Hwang, S., Altshuler, L. L., Elman, S., Zuckerbrow-Miller, J., & Korenman, S. G. (2003). Depression in women with polycystic ovary syndrome: Clinical and biochemical correlates. *Journal of Affective Disorders, 74*, 299–304.

Roaldset, J. O., Linaker, O. M., & Bjørkly, S. (2012). Predictive validity of the MINI suicidal scale for self-harm in acute psychiatry: A prospective study of the first year after discharge. *Archives of Suicide Research, 16*(4), 287–302.

Salehifar, D., Lotfi, R., & Ramezani Tehrani, F. (2016). The comparative study of depression in women with polycystic ovary syndrome and control group. *Iranian Journal of Endocrinology and Metabolism, 18*(3), 180–186.

Scaruffi, E., Gambineri, A., Cattaneo, S., Turra, J., Vettor, R., & Mioni, R. (2014). Personality and psychiatric disorders in women affected by polycystic ovary syndrome. *Frontiers in Endocrinology, 5*, 185.

Sheehan, D. V., Lecrubier, Y., Sheehan, K. H., Amorim, P., Janavs, J., Weiller, E., … Dunbar, G. C. (1998). The Mini-International Neuropsychiatric Interview (MINI): The development and validation of a structured diagnostic psychiatric interview for DSM-IV and ICD-10. *The Journal of Clinical Psychiatry*.

Soyupek, F., Guney, M., Eris, S., Cerci, S., Yildiz, S., & Mungan, T. (2008). Evaluation of hand functions in women with polycystic ovary syndrome. *Gynecological Endocrinology, 24*, 571–575.

Spielberger, C. D. (1995). *State-trait depression scales (Form X-1)*. Palo Alto: Mind Garden.

Stapinska-Syniec, A., Grabowska, K., Szpotanska-Sikorska, M., & Pietrzak, B. (2018). Depression, sexual satisfaction, and other psychological issues in women with polycystic ovary syndrome. *Gynecological Endocrinology, 34*(7), 597–600.

Stunkard, A. J., Faith, A. S., & Allison, K. C. (2003). Depression and obesity. *Biological Psychiatry, 54*, 330–337.

Tabachnick, B. G., & Fidell, L. S. (2006). *Using multivariate statistics* (5th international Ed.). Boston: Pearson.

Teede, H. J., Misso, M. L., Deeks, A. A., Moran, L. J., Stuckey, B. G., Wong, J. L., … Costello, M. F. (2011). Assessment and management of polycystic ovary syndrome: Summary of an evidence-based guideline. *The Medical Journal of Australia, 195*(6), 65.

Wake, D. J., Strand, M., Rask, E., Westerbacka, J., Livingstone, D. E., Soderberg, S., … Walker, B. R. (2007). Intra-adipose sex steroid metabolism and body fat distribution in idiopathic human obesity. *Clinical Endocrinology, 66*, 440–446.

Weiner, C. L., Primeau, M., & Ehrmann, D. A. (2004). Androgens & mood dysfunction in women: Comparison of women with PCOS to healthy controls. *Psychosomatic Medicine, 66*, 356–362.

Young, R., & Sinclair, R. (1998). Hirsutes. I: Diagnosis. *The Australasian Journal of Dermatology, 39*, 24–28.

Zehra, S., Arif, A., Anjum, N., Azhar, A., & Qureshi, M. (2015). Depression and anxiety in women with polycystic ovary syndrome from Pakistan. *Life Science Journal, 12*(3s), 1–4.

Zhao, Y., & Qiao, J. (2013). Ethnic differences in the phenotypic expression of polycystic ovary syndrome. *Steroids, 78*(8), 755–760.

Zigmond, A. S., & Snaith, R. P. (1983). The hospital anxiety and depression scale. *Acta Psychiatrica Scandinavica, 67*(6), 361–370.

3

Anxiety and Other Psychological Issues in PCOS

Abstract Anxiety is usually seen as less important than depression in polycystic ovary syndrome (PCOS), but this chapter shows that the secondary status of anxiety is misplaced. Firstly, anxiety is probably a more clinically significant issue than depression in PCOS. Secondly, the causes of anxiety are probably more complex than they are for depression in PCOS, involving a greater number of psychobiological pathways. Thirdly, there is the interesting question of how much anxiety and stress can be a cause as well as a product of PCOS. This chapter also examines the impact of PCOS on quality of life (QoL), and describes some of the new and lesser-researched psychological issues that might be associated with PCOS, such as autism spectrum disorder (ASD).

Keywords Anxiety • Quality of life (QoL) • Hypoglycaemia • Neuroticism • Autism spectrum disorder (ASD)

© The Author(s) 2019
J. A. Barry, *Psychological Aspects of Polycystic Ovary Syndrome*,
https://doi.org/10.1007/978-3-030-30290-0_3

Introduction

This chapter will mainly explore the role of anxiety in polycystic ovary syndrome (PCOS). It will also look at some of the other psychological conditions that have been associated with PCOS, but with less frequency than depression and anxiety. Two anxiety-related topics will be discussed in other chapters: the important impact of hypoglycaemia on anxiety will be discussed in Chap. 5 (on insulin) and the relationship between fertility and anxiety will be discussed in Chap. 6.

The distinction between anxiety and depression is potentially important in PCOS because, as I describe in this chapter, it is likely that the underlying cause of anxiety is different than that for depression. As we saw in the previous chapter, the cause of depression in PCOS is most likely to be a reaction to the troubling symptoms of PCOS. However, the cause of anxiety in PCOS is likely to be somewhat different. Both problems have their root in elevated testosterone (which itself is rooted in insulin resistance—see Chap. 5), but for depression the cause is hypothesised to be circulating levels of testosterone which cause unpleasant symptoms, and for anxiety the cause is hypothesised to be the organisational effect of prenatal testosterone which programme for the development of insulin resistance, and therefore hypoglycaemia, in the adult. These two different pathways are both indirect, and both explained in full in Chap. 7, but in the present chapter we will just focus on the immediate causes of anxiety in PCOS.

This chapter will also give an overview of other psychological issues that have been linked with PCOS; this section will be relatively short, reflecting the relative paucity of information on these issues. Note that although there are links to some conditions that sound rather serious (e.g. autism spectrum disorder), readers should be aware that the evidence for these issues is limited, and tends to indicate relatively mild problems (e.g. Asperger syndrome rather than autism).

Measurement of Anxiety

The Hospital Anxiety and Depression Scale (HADS; Zigmond and Snaith 1983) is sometimes used in PCOS research. This scale measures the state of anxiety and depression in medical outpatients by asking them to rate 14 statements, seven on anxiety and seven on depression on a 4-point scale. An example of an item from the Anxiety scale is 'I feel tense or "wound up"'. An example from the depression scale is 'I still enjoy the things I used to enjoy'. The response options are 'Most of the time; A lot of the time; From time to time/ occasionally; Not at all'. Scores of 8–10 indicate a mild problem; 11–14 a moderate problem; and 15–21 a clinical problem.

Validated measures—those that have had their psychometric properties evaluated—should be used in research. At a minimum, this ensures that the findings are reasonably valid (they measure what you think they are measuring) and reliable (they will give the same scores under similar circumstances). Even if a large sample size is used, the findings are in doubt if validated instruments are not used. For example, Barnard et al. (2007) found that 29% of women with PCOS reported experiencing anxiety compared to under 8% of healthy controls. However, this was done using an unpublished measure of anxiety, which seems to have underestimated anxiety, which is probably—including mild levels—around 63% in PCOS and 29% in healthy women (see section below 'How severe is anxiety in PCOS', with data based on Cooney et al. 2017).

Sometimes anxiety seems an afterthought to depression in studies of PCOS, as if one was a less important aspect of the other. It should be recognised, however, that they are separate constructs, albeit ones that tend to be correlated and often co-occur. For example, a woman with PCOS might feel both depressed (feels sad because she thinks she will always be obese) and anxious (worries that people at an upcoming social event will notice her facial hair). However, just because the two experiences co-occur doesn't mean they are the same thing, or that they have the same cause. So although the measures tend to be strongly correlated the lack of a *total* correlation ($r = 1.0$) is a clue to the fact that they are distinct constructs. An example of this is that Xie et al. (2012) found that although the HADS anxiety and depression subscales correlated strongly in pain patients ($r = 0.64$), this leaves around a third (0.36) of scoring that is not in common to the two subscales. This suggests that although there might be an underlying common factor to anxiety and depression, for example, general psychological distress (or perhaps neuroticism—see section below), some part of what is being measured by each scale is different to what is being measured by the other.

A character trait is a consistent pattern of thinking, feeling, and behaving (Pervin 1994). Some scales differentiate between depressed state (a feeling that might come or go depending on the situation) or depressed state (a feeling that endures across most situations). An example is the State-Trait Anxiety Inventory (STAI; Spielberger et al. 1999).

'Anxiety', 'stress', and 'distress' are often used somewhat interchangeably. More specific definitions can be found, but in this chapter I will use the term somewhat loosely, as is usual in PCOS research, though I hope the terms make sense in context. In general, *anxiety* will refer to a measured state of worry; 'stress' is a stressor (something causing stress) or an experience of some level of distress; and distress will mean a state of anxiety or discomfort whether measured or not. I will sometimes make the usual distinction between psychological stress/distress and physiological stress/distress, although these terms might be seen to separately impact cognition (thoughts), affect (feelings), behaviour, and physiology.

Experiencing stress is fairly normal in everyday life, and usually only turns into a problem if it becomes enduring. Thus we talk about acute or chronic stress and so on, and although in PCOS much of the anxiety/stress/distress can be thought of as chronic, much of the research in this book is cross-sectional so it is difficult to say how chronic the stress is, unless that has been identified specifically in a study.

Anxiety and Stress in PCOS

We have known for a long time (e.g. Monzani et al. 1994) that anxiety tends to be higher in women with PCOS compared to healthy women. Several studies have also found that women with PCOS often experience raised anxiety levels (e.g. Månsson et al. 2008; Elsenbruch et al. 2003; McCook 2002; Greiner et al. 2005; and Keegan et al. 2003). Although anxiety levels may sometimes be only mildly raised in PCOS compared to other women, the difference is statistically significant and potentially clinically significant, for reasons discussed below.

What Causes Anxiety in PCOS?

We saw in the previous chapter that depression in PCOS is most likely to be related to distressing symptoms related to PCOS, such as obesity and hirsutism. It would be easy to presume that in a similar way anxiety in PCOS is caused by the perception of the PCOS symptoms, but would this be correct? Although some authors have found that obesity contributes to psychological distress in PCOS (e.g. Elsenbruch et al. 2006), the answer is slightly more complex, because while it is likely that symptoms contribute to the anxiety in PCOS, there is also evidence that anxiety in PCOS may be rooted more so in insulin resistance than is the case for depression.

Does Anxiety/Stress Cause PCOS?

PCOS is a complex condition, and in no ways more complex that the relationship between anxiety and PCOS symptoms. We now enter controversial waters in addressing the suggestion that distress might actually be a contributor to the symptoms of PCOS, or might even be the cause of PCOS. Stress causes increased visceral fat and inflammation and can, as Farrell and Antoni (2010) put it, trigger 'a negative spiral leading to greater insulin resistance and subsequent hyperandrogenism, exacerbating clinical symptoms such as infertility, acne, and hirsutism, and possibly negative affect as well' (Farrell and Antoni 2010, p. 1568). So although stress doesn't cause PCOS, for women who already have PCOS, stress potentially can exacerbate the symptoms.

It is well established that in healthy men and women, stress activates the adrenal glands via the hypothalamic-pituitary-adrenal axis (HPA) (Reiche et al. 2004). What is less well known is that healthy women produce roughly 25% of their testosterone via bioconversion of adrenal androgens, mainly androstenedione and dehydroepiandrosterone sulphate (DHEAS), created in the adrenal glands (Burger 2002). Balikci et al. (2014) found that Beck's Anxiety Inventory scores were significantly correlated with DHEAS in PCOS ($r = 0.44$, $p < 0.001$). Putting this information together, we can see that the level of stress a woman experiences in her daily life may potentially exacerbate her PCOS symptoms. However, research suggests that women with PCOS take this mechanism to another level.

There is evidence that women with PCOS show a stronger HPA response to a stressor than healthy women. In a small but groundbreaking study of stress in PCOS, Modell et al. (1990) found that although a baseline measure of trait anxiety was similar between two groups of women, 13 with PCOS and 13 controls, after undertaking mental arithmetic problems, state anxiety and various hormones were disrupted in women with PCOS compared to the controls. Using the Stroop task as a stressor, Gallinelli et al. (2000) found that cortisol levels became higher in the PCOS group compared to controls. Benson et al. (2009) compared 32 women with PCOS to 32 BMI- and age-matched controls in their HPA responsivity to a stress-inducing public speaking task. They found that in the PCOS group, ACTH, cortisol, and heart rate all became significantly higher than controls in response to the task. Use of metformin did not have an impact on these differences.

With a sample of 18 women with PCOS and 12 healthy control women, Greiner et al. (2005) found anxiety was significantly higher in PCOS, as measured on Goldberg's General Health Questionnaire (GHQ-30). Interestingly, although the circadian cortisol pattern was not different between groups, a significantly lower percentage of the PCOS group secreted low levels of urinary cortisol, and a significantly higher percentage of the PCOS group were unable to suppress cortisol below 1 µg/mL in response to an overnight 1 mg dexamethasone suppressor test; both of these results are indicators of increased sympathetic tone in the PCOS group. The authors conclude that the biochemical alterations caused the anxiety seen in the PCOS group, but how strong this relationship might be was not explored—the authors did not statistically correlate the psychological and biochemical outcomes.

Interestingly, the 5% or so of women with PCOS who are lean may be even more prone than women with a typical PCOS presentation to disturbances in the hypothalamic-pituitary-adrenal axis, and it has even been suggested that hypothalamic dysfunction is implicated in the pathogenesis of lean PCOS (Goyal and Dawood 2017).

In their review of PCOS and stress, Eggers and Kirchengast (2001) suggest that PCOS may be a cause of distress to the individual (due to symptoms) as well as be exacerbated by psychosocial stressors (e.g. major life events). However, sometimes information, on the internet or mainstream media goes a step (or a leap) further, suggesting things like 'the main causes of PCOS are high levels of stress & poor lifestyle' (Moss 2016). This type of suggestion is probably overstating the case, though as we can see there is certainly a credible mechanism connecting stress and PCOS.

How Severe Is Anxiety in PCOS?

The meta-analysis by Barry et al. (2011b) found that the most commonly used measure of anxiety was the STAI-S, used in five of the six included studies, and the norm anxiety score for women of this age group is 36.2 (Spielberger et al. 1999). In these five studies it was found that for women with PCOS anxiety levels were statistically significantly higher (Hedges' $g = 0.46$, $p < 0.0005$) than in controls. As with the depression scores seen in the previous chapter, the mean anxiety scores indicated mild anxiety in the women with PCOS (40.7) and none in the controls (34.6). A relatively large study in Australia using the HADS found a similar pattern of scoring in 177 women with PCOS and 109 controls (Deeks et al. 2011). However, even though the elevations of anxiety in PCOS are often mild, it is worth bearing in mind what we know about HPA reactivity in PCOS (see previous section), which means that even a modest increase in anxiety might be of clinical significance because of the potential to exacerbate the symptoms of PCOS. In some cases anxiety might be severe enough to warrant professional attention, and this might possibly be especially so in lean women with PCOS (Goyal and Dawood 2017) though more research is needed on this relatively small subgroup.

The meta-analysis by Cooney et al. (2017) reported that the prevalence of anxiety in PCOS was 41.9% and 8.5% in the control groups of the nine included studies, and that odds of having anxiety symptoms was five times higher in PCOS, and moderate and severe anxiety symptoms were six times higher. Although these odds are higher than for depression (see Chap. 2) what was the actual prevalence of moderate and severe anxiety symptoms in each group?

Of the 30 studies cited in their Supplementary Table III, 11 reported anxiety rates, and 5 identified the specific level of anxiety (mild, moderate or severe). Using this subset of data, the mean rates of mild anxiety were PCOS = 20.5 %, controls = 19.0%; of moderate anxiety were PCOS = 34.3%, controls = 7.6%; and of severe anxiety were PCOS = 8.6%, controls = 1.7%. Using these data, the rates for moderate and severe anxiety combined are PCOS = 44.9%, controls = 9.3%, which are higher than the rates of moderate to severe depression (25% in PCOS and 6.5% in controls) seen in the previous chapter.

Neuroticism

Neuroticism is a psychological term that describes a character trait that combines a fluctuating mix of various negative states, mainly anxiety, depression, and anger. It is often measured as a subscale of the Eysenck Personality Questionnaire (EPQ; Eysenck and Eysenck 1987). Examples of the items are 'Does your mood often go up and down?' 'Are your feelings easily hurt?' 'Would you call yourself tense or highly strung?' 'Do you often feel lonely?' and 'Are you often troubled about feelings of guilt?' Eysenck and Eysenck suggest that neuroticism is caused by lability of the autonomic nervous system (ANS) and predisposes a person to cope poorly with stressful events. This fits well with Farrell and Antoni's (2010) observation that women with PCOS have an exaggerated SNS response (sympathetic nervous system, the 'fight or flight' part of the ANS) to stress, and this response would contribute to elevated adrenal products, such as cortisol and DHEAS, and chronic inflammation. Although the term 'neurotic' has developed a somewhat pejorative connotation in popular usage, this construct is useful because it captures quite well a lot of the mood issues and stress seen in PCOS.

Neuroticism was first identified in PCOS in 2011 (Barry et al. 2011a), and although few studies have focused on neuroticism since then, a large twin study has found a genetic link between depression, neuroticism, and

PCOS (Cesta 2017). The link with anxiety is established too, though in a non-PCOS study; in a twin study of over 4000 pairs, Hettema et al. (2004) found a strong correlation between generalised anxiety disorder and neuroticism. Because there is very little research on neuroticism in PCOS, it is necessary to assess some of the research on non-PCOS populations. Previous research on non-PCOS women had linked neuroticism to three conditions that are associated with PCOS: hirsutism, cardiovascular disease (CVD), and fertility problems. Barth et al. (1993) studied 69 hirsute patients and found high neuroticism scores, as measured on the EPQ. None were identified as having PCOS, and the authors did not compare the results to a control group but the mean score of 14.6 ± 4.0 is roughly 25% higher than the norm for women (Eysenck and Eysenck 1987). It is also higher than the neuroticism scores for obese non-PCOS women (Faith et al. 2001).

In women without PCOS, and men too, neuroticism is associated with health outcomes. In a 21-year prospective survey of 5424 adults in the general population of men and women, Shipley et al. (2007) found that after controlling for gender, age, social class, education, smoking, alcohol consumption, physical activity, and health, high neuroticism scores were significantly related to mortality from cardiovascular disease. Verhaak et al. (2005) studied 187 women who had recently failed to conceive after one treatment cycle with either in vitro fertilisation (IVF) or Intracytoplasmic Sperm Injection (ICSI). The causes of infertility were 33% idiopathic (i.e. of spontaneous or unknown cause), 22% female causes, 35% male causes, and 10% a combination of male and female causes. The mean age was 34.3 years, and the mean duration of fertility problems was 3.3 years. Measures included the EPQ, STAI, and Beck's Depression Inventory (BDI). The infertile women scored slightly below the norm for neuroticism at baseline (before failing the first cycle): 4.7 (SD 3.0) versus 5.72 (SD 2.91). However after the failed cycle there was a significant increase in anxiety and depression ($p < 0.001$ for both). The largest correlation between the change in the anxiety score from baseline to time 2 was for neuroticism ($p < 0.001$). The change in depression was also correlated with neuroticism ($p < 0.001$). Multiple regression showed that baseline neuroticism scores were the best predictors of anxiety and depression after the failed cycle.

The above studies demonstrate that in non-PCOS populations, neuroticism has proven links with conditions that are associated with PCOS: hirsutism, CVD, and infertility. Because neuroticism could be a key underlying factor in the psychology and biology of PCOS, further research on this topic is recommended.

Quality of Life in PCOS

In contrast to narrower constructs such as anxiety and depression, health-related quality of life (HRQoL, or HRQL) is defined as 'a multidimensional concept that encompasses physical, emotional and social aspects associated with a specific disease or its treatment' (Jones et al. 2007, p. 15). The concept of quality of life (QoL) is slightly broader, encompassing non-health issues, and will mainly be used in this section. Many of the studies below focus on various psychological aspects of PCOS, and, although not all are QoL, it might be considered that QoL is implicitly measured to some extent in studies of anxiety and depression, not least because there is some evidence that the three constructs are related (Lipton et al. 2006; Barnard et al. 2007).

One of the most widely used measures of HRQoL in medicine is the Short Form 36 (known as the SF-36), a widely used generic scale (Ware et al. 1992). It has 36 items and eight dimensions (vitality, physical functioning, bodily pain, general health perceptions, physical role functioning, emotional role functioning, social role functioning, and mental health). Higher scores indicate better QoL. A measure designed for women with PCOS is the polycystic ovary syndrome questionnaire (PCOSQ) (Cronin et al. 1998). The initial validation included only 100 women, and a later correction was needed—with the addition of an item on acne suggested by Jones et al. (2004). The PCOSQ measures five dimensions: emotions, face/body hair, acne, infertility, and weight and menstrual problems. (QoL for infertility is discussed in Chap. 6.) The PCOSQ has been used in many studies of PCOS. For example, Greenwood et al. (2018) found that depressed women with PCOS reported worse QoL for mood, weight, menstrual problems, infertility, and body hair.

A more recent measurement tool is the PCOS Quality of Life Questionnaire (PCOSQOL) (Williams et al. 2018). This has subscales for the general impact of PCOS, infertility, hirsutism, and mood. It does not have a subscale for obesity for the statistical reason that all of the items relating to body weight failed to load on to a single factor. Perhaps the findings reflect the population sampled from—UK PCOS groups on Facebook—which may have contained a higher proportion of women who were more unconcerned with body weight than usually seen in studies of PCOS, though the absence of a weight subscale could make generalising from studies using the PCOSQOL a challenge when it comes to body weight issues.

QoL scales are not primarily about psychology, and tend to focus more on other dimensions impacted in illness than the psychological or emotional dimensions. Indeed there is some evidence that greater sensitivity is needed towards psychological/emotional aspects in QoL scales for PCOS in order to increase sensitivity to changes due to treatment interventions (Barry et al. 2018). Curiously, none of the current QoL scales include items on sleep, an oversight which should be remedied in future PCOS QoL questionnaire developments.

In their review of QoL measures of PCOS, Moghadam et al. (2018) suggest that QoL in PCOS should be measured either with the PCOSQ or with the PCOSQ in tandem with the SF-36 in order to capture both specific issues in PCOS and general HRQoL issues. I would suggest using both because the findings of the PCOSQ can be compared to the scores of other studies of PCOS using that instrument, or measure the impact on PCOS symptoms of an intervention pre and post, whereas the SF-36 allows you to compare scores of women with PCOS to scores of non-PCOS women in order to see the general health impact of PCOS compared to other conditions.

A study that emphasises the fact that PCOS is a difficult condition to have—and more than just a physical condition—found that although women with PCOS scored similarly for physical problems to women with diabetes, epilepsy, back pain, and asthma, they scored much lower (i.e. had worse QoL) on the mental health dimension, by about 20% (Coffey et al. 2006). Another study emphasising the relatively distressing nature of PCOS was conducted by Mącik (2016) who found that QoL can be worse in PCOS than QoL in women post mastectomy.

Quality of Life and Obesity

In their review of the QoL literature on PCOS, Jones et al. (2007) found that weight problems had the greatest negative impact on quality of life, a view echoed in the review by Moghadam et al. (2018). Research shows that issues with weight begin in adolescence when the symptoms of PCOS manifest and continue into adulthood. Using the CHQ-CF87 (Child Health Questionnaire) Trent et al. (2005) found that 97 adolescents with PCOS had worse HRQoL for weight issues than 186 healthy adolescent girls. McCook et al. (2005) found that weight was the main PCOSQ domain affecting adult women (mean age 30.4 ± 5.5). McCook et al. (2005) and Hahn et al. (2005) found a significant correlation between QoL weight scores and BMI suggesting that a higher BMI is associated with a worse quality of life regarding weight.

Jones et al. (2007) point out that in the PCOS literature, BMI does not necessarily affect QoL domains other than weight (e.g. McCook et al. 2005). This is interesting because Wake et al. (2007) found that obesity contributes to higher androgen levels via the decrease in aromatase activity in adipose tissue, so we should expect that BMI has a global impact on features affected by testosterone, that is, the other PCOSQ domains of acne, hirsutism, fertility, and (indirectly) emotions. However the fact that a direct correlation between BMI and other QoL variables does not always exist indicates the complexity of the interrelationships between the many variables involved in PCOS. Psychological factors may impact a relationship between BMI and QoL; for example, good general coping skills might reduce the QoL impact of BMI. A measurement issue that might contribute to the lack of direct BMI/QoL correlation is the possibility that the waist-to-hip ratio (WHR) is a better measure of android or central obesity than BMI (Carranza-Lira et al. 2006); thus, the WHR might be more sensitive to QoL issues than BMI. Central obesity—weight gain around the stomach rather than hips—is more typically seen in men because one of the causes is elevated androgens. Perhaps because of the association with men, it is considered unattractive in women in many cultures (Brown 1991).

Overall there is at least some evidence that HRQoL is improved by weight loss in both women with PCOS (Hahn et al. 2006) and the general population (Kolotkin et al. 2001).

Quality of Life and Hirsutism

Hirsutism can cause distress to women with PCOS (see section on *Social Avoidance* below). Clayton et al. (2005) found that laser treatment for facial hirsutism improved HRQoL and HADS anxiety and depression scores compared to a control group. Using the World Health Organization Quality of Life instrument, brief version (WHOQoL-BREF) Kumarapeli et al. (2008) found that hirsutism was the main cause of psychological distress in 146 women with PCOS. In contrast Keegan et al. (2003) did not find a significant correlation between distress and hirsutism in their study of 53 women with PCOS. In fact, there is little consistent relationship between objective measures of hirsutism and QoL for hirsutism; while McCook et al. (2005) found the expected correlation, Trent et al. (2002) and Guyatt et al. (2004) did not. The sometimes inconsistent relationship between objective versus subjective measures is a recurring theme in QoL research and hirsutism can be difficult to assess even using the most popular measure, the Ferriman-Gallwey assessment, partly due to the ethnic differences in hair growth (Karimah and Hestiantoro 2016). However, when the complex worlds of psychology and biology collide, we should expect these correlations to be complicated. For example, in a simplified world, you would expect there to be a strong correlation between testosterone and hirsutism, but in fact the correlation between testosterone and hirsutism is relatively weak; $r = 0.24$ at best, according to Legro et al. (2010). This lets us know that androgens other than testosterone—especially dihydrotestosterone (DHT) but possibly also androgens—are more causal of hirsutism than is testosterone. That is probably why even when testosterone decreases in PCOS, hirsutism does not reduce significantly (Palomba et al. 2007).

QoL and Sleep

Sleep difficulties have not been widely recognised in PCOS until the past few years. For example, the Jones et al. PCOSQ questionnaire didn't include any items for sleep. Little surprise then that obstructive sleep apnoea (OSA) may go undiagnosed in PCOS, even though the review by

Kahal et al. (2017) found that it is more common in women with PCOS than other women. OSA, like PCOS, is associated with insulin resistance, depression, and fatigue. OSA is also associated with increased blood pressure. OSA occurs more so in women (and men) who are obese, though in PCOS sleep disturbance cannot be fully explained by obesity.

In the past decade sleep disturbance has increasingly been the subject of interesting research. Lin et al. (2017) conducted a longitudinal study from two to eight years using a Taiwanese database. They found over twice the rate of OSA in 4595 women with PCOS compared to 4595 age-matched female controls, independent of obesity and demographic characteristics. Using the same Taiwanese database, Hung et al. (2014) found that women with PCOS were 50% more likely to be diagnosed with a sleeping disorder than age-matched controls. Moran et al. (2015) found that problems falling asleep were twice as common in their Australian study of 87 women with PCOS and 637 female controls, independent of age, BMI, or level of depression. However difficulty in remaining asleep appeared to be related to BMI and depression.

The results from clinic-based studies have generally been supportive of the community-based studies. Though these clinic studies tend to be small in sample size (~12 to 50 participants), the findings replicate reasonably well (e.g. Fogel et al. 2001; Suri et al. 2016; Tasali 2006, 2008). One of the larger studies (Franik et al. 2016) compared 95 women with PCOS to 130 controls and found that clinically significant insomnia was three to ten times higher in women with PCOS, depending on the measure used. Underlining the importance of the measure used, Álvarez-Blasco et al. (2010) chose the Nottingham Health Profile (NHP) to assess sleep in 32 women with PCOS and 72 healthy controls, but found no effect of either PCOS status or weight. The NHP is a general questionnaire, and it is very possible that had Álvarez-Blasco et al. used a questionnaire with other assessment methods that were more sleep-orientated, this might have been better able to detect sleep issues.

A review by Fernandez et al. (2018) suggests that the cause of sleep disturbance in PCOS is complex, probably involving the impact of HPA problems (as noted above) on secretion of the sleep hormone melatonin. Sleep disturbance can lead to a vicious cycle of low mood and dysfunctional coping (e.g. drinking alcohol), which exacerbate insomnia. This is a particularly vicious cycle in PCOS, because poor sleep is associated with increased risk of type 2 diabetes, thereby increasing distressing PCOS symptoms.

Social Avoidance

There is evidence that from an early age women with PCOS may have interpersonal difficulties. Manlove et al. (2008) found that compared to controls, women with PCOS reported that as children they felt less cared for by both their mother and father, and resented or disliked their brother more. This same group reported less sociability in adolescence, and reported more time spent reading and babysitting, and less time playing sports or dating boys.

Månsson et al. (2008) found higher rates of social phobia in women with PCOS compared to age-matched controls. Basirat et al. (2018) found that 120 infertile women with PCOS had more difficulty expressing their feelings (alexithymia) than 120 infertile controls. Kitzinger and Willmott (2002) found that women with PCOS were sometimes in despair about their appearance, with hirsutism making some women feel 'freakish', and similar sentiments regarding hirsutism were expressed in interviews with 21 Danish women with PCOS (Pfister and Rømer 2017). Hirsutism, even in women who don't have PCOS, can cause social and emotional stress (Barth et al. 1993), and more anxiety and social fears than in non-hirsute women (Sonino et al. 1993). Emeksiz et al. (2018) found that hirsutism was associated with panic disorder in adolescent women with PCOS. Açmaz et al. (2013) compared 86 women with PCOS to 47 healthy control women. The group that showed the most problems, including socialising, were those hirsute women with oligomenorrhea. These women scored badly in terms of physical functioning, physical role function, pain, social functioning, emotional role function, and emotional well-being.

One might speculate that adding to hirsutism the other problems of PCOS might make socialising additionally uncomfortable, but the evidence is mixed regarding the degree to which other PCOS symptoms cause social unease. Using the SF-36, Hahn et al. (2006) found that although obesity worsened physical QoL, social and emotional QoL were not related to obesity. Coffey et al. (2006) found that 22 women with PCOS scored worse than 96 healthy controls on all PCOSQ and SF-36 subscales, apart from physical and social functioning. In contrast, Keegan et al. (2003) did not find women with PCOS scored higher than normative levels on the Social Avoidance and Distress scale.

Overall, while there is some evidence of a negative impact of PCOS on social QoL, the evidence is mixed. BMI does not appear to be the root cause, and it seems that women with hirsutism suffer the greatest fears socially. The relationship between social avoidance and PCOS symptoms is most likely indirect; Himelein and Thatcher (2006a) suggest that body dissatisfaction might be a cause of anxiety and depression in PCOS, and; Himelein and Thatcher (2006b) suggest depression causes social avoidance.

Body Dissatisfaction in PCOS

It is especially unfortunate that the symptoms of PCOS emerge at the time when looking attractive often becomes especially important in a young woman's life. Self-esteem seems to be related to QoL issues in PCOS. de Niet et al. (2010) recruited 480 women with PCOS from a clinic in Holland between 1991 and 2006, and found reduced self-esteem and body satisfaction compared to the general population. Pastore et al. (2011) compared 96 women with PCOS to a community cohort of 94 matched by BMI category. They found that for all women, depression was positively correlated with dissatisfaction with not only physical appearance, but aspects of fitness that are not generally visible, for example, stamina and agility. This suggests that body dissatisfaction in PCOS is not just about outward appearance, but also about how fit and healthy one feels is also important. Supporting this hypothesis, in their study of 300 women with PCOS in Iran, Bazarganipour et al. (2013) found that infertile women had significantly lower levels of self-esteem and body satisfaction. There are possibly cultural differences too in how body weight is perceived; Alur-Gupta et al. (2019) found that BMI was correlated with anxiety in white women but not black women.

Other Possible Psychological Issues in PCOS

Firstly, a word of caution regarding the use of psychiatric scales with non-psychiatric patients; this may result in 'false positive' diagnosis of psychiatric conditions. Scaruffi et al. (2014) used the Millon Clinical Multiaxial Inventory-III (MCMI-III) on 60 women with PCOS recruited from non-psychiatric medical centres, and Elsenbruch et al. (2006) used the Symptom Checklist 90-Revised (SCL-90-R) with 143 women with PCOS. Both studies found elevations on various subscales (though Elsenbruch et al. found that this was largely accounted for by BMI in the PCOS group), and although these findings are of interest, we should be cautious not to take the findings as equivalent to a psychiatric diagnosis.

In an epidemiological analysis of a Swedish register, Cesta et al. (2016) found evidence of a wide range of psychiatric issues related to PCOS, including schizophrenia, bipolar disorder, bulimia, autism spectrum disorder (ASD), tics, and personality disorders. They concluded that there may be shared genetic factors between PCOS and psychiatric disorders. These findings may have highlighted some conditions that have been previously overlooked, and may prove to be of clinical significance. Follow-up research is needed.

Cesta et al. (2016) identified all women diagnosed with PCOS on Swedish national registers between 1990 and 2013 (n = 24,385) and their full-siblings (n = 25,921). These were matched to people from the general population, and their full-siblings. They presented their results both as *crude* ORs and as the ORs *adjusted* (AORs) for psychiatric comorbidities. This adjustment is made to control for the confounding impact of relevant variables. For example, in seeing whether women with PCOS are more likely to commit suicide than non-PCOS women, the analysis makes sure that the presence or number or psychiatric issues isn't different in the PCOS and non-PCOS groups. This is done in order that we are not comparing, for example, the suicide risk in a woman with PCOS with mild depression to a healthy control woman with major depression and schizophrenia. Although Cesta et al. found a small increase in suicide when using the crude ORs (OR = 1.41), the adjusted ORs indicated no elevated risk of suicide in PCOS (See discussion in Chap. 2). Cesta et al.

also found that after adjusting for comorbid psychiatric disorders, women with PCOS were significantly more likely to have tics (AOR = 1.65), anxious or fearful personality disorders (AOR = 1.60), ASD (AOR = 1.55), bipolar disorder (AOR = 1.41), anxiety disorders (AOR = 1.37), schizophrenia (AOR = 1.36), depressive disorders (AOR = 1.25), and bulimia (AOR = 1.21).

Some findings of interest were that anxiety disorders were more of a risk than depressive disorders, which is interesting, firstly, because this reflects the findings above and in Chap. 2, and, secondly, because anxiety is less often measured in studies of PCOS. The finding regarding tics is novel. Many people will be unfamiliar with tics in a psychological sense: these are sudden movements (e.g. blinking, shrugging) or sounds (e.g. humming, throat clearing, or shouting a word) that happen repeatedly and uncontrollably (American Psychiatric Association 2013). Although it is known that tics can be part of ASD, this analysis controlled for the presence of comorbidities (such as ASD).

They also found increased risk of women with PCOS being diagnosed with personality disorders, although a weakness of the study design is that the specific type of personality disorder could not be identified, except by their general category, or 'cluster'. The highest risk (AOR = 1.60) was in cluster C, a category of disorders consisting of 'Avoidant personality disorder: pervasive feelings of social inhibition and inadequacy, extreme sensitivity to negative evaluation; Dependent personality disorder: pervasive psychological need to be cared for by other people; and Obsessive-compulsive personality disorder: characterized by rigid conformity to rules, perfectionism, and control to the point of satisfaction and exclusion of leisurely activities and friendships (distinct from obsessive-compulsive disorder)' (Mayo Clinic 2019). It is easy to see how women with PCOS might, by virtue of being sensitive about their symptoms, show avoidant behaviours, and by virtue of having a medical condition feel the need to be cared for. However, getting a diagnosis of this kind means that these behaviours would need to be fairly obvious and persistent. Unfortunately the analysis does not show which specific disorder(s) apply to PCOS.

The second highest risk (AOR = 1.49) was in cluster A, a category of disorders consisting of paranoid, schizoid, and schizotypal personality disorders. These are characterised by being suspicious of others and being very uncomfortable in social situations. The least high risk (AOR = 1.27), though still statistically significant, was cluster B, consisting of antisocial, borderline, histrionic, and narcissistic personality disorders. This cluster is characterised by dramatic, overly emotional, or unpredictable thinking or behaviour. There is little previous research on this topic, but these findings give some support to Kawamura et al. (2011) who found genetic similarities between PCOS and borderline personality disorder with comorbid major depression.

Previous evidence of psychiatric disorders in PCOS has been relatively weak (e.g. Sahingöz et al. 2013) but the findings of Cesta et al., being based on a large register, are much stronger. However, as impressive as this study is, there are weaknesses. Firstly, data for BMI and insulin resistance were not in the register, and although there are problems with controlling for variables that are systematically different between groups (discussed in Chap. 2), it was unfortunate that the BMI of women in this study was not identified. If there were data for BMI we could have at least looked at simple correlations between these variables and outcomes such as depression, especially because Elsenbruch et al. (2006) found that many of the psychiatric issues that appeared higher in PCOS were accounted for to a large degree by BMI. Secondly, the effect sizes were relatively small in many cases, and are of statistical significance with the help of the very large sample size. Even for the largest effect size (for tics) the adjusted odds ratio was 1.65 (95% CI, 1.10–2.47); in other words, women with PCOS have a 65% higher risk of having tics than other women. This might sound like a lot, but not so much if understood as meaning women with PCOS have a higher chance, but not twice the chance, of experiencing a tic. In perspective, Cesta et al. found that having tics was a rare event, occurring in only 0.1% of their PCOS sample (24 out of 24,385 women), which was roughly double the rate in the control group.

Lastly, it should be noted that the psychiatric conditions are not identified by diagnosis in all cases. The register is large because it combines several nationwide longitudinal registers, and although the data is useful for research purposes, and some of the labels will indicate a diagnosis by a psychiatrist, in general the psychiatric labels cannot be considered fully valid. However this is a weakness of many databases, and does not negate the potential importance of the findings of the excellent work of Cesta et al. (2016).

Bipolar Disorder

Cesta et al. (2016) found a 41% increased chance of bipolar disorder in 24,385 women with PCOS, independent of other psychiatric morbidities, but there is some debate and confusion over whether bipolar disorder is truly related to PCOS, mainly based on how much the association is because a medication used to treat bipolar disorder (valproate) might also induce PCOS. Although Scaruffi et al. (2014) found only around 2% bipolar disorder in women with PCOS, other authors have found higher rates, for example, Klipstein and Goldberg (2006) who found a rate of around 27% bipolar disorder in women with PCOS with no history of valproate use. A laboratory study found support for a mechanism that might cause the bipolar/PCOS link (Nelson-DeGrave et al. 2004), but although Rasgon et al. (2005) found high rates of menstrual irregularities in women taking valproate, they did not find increased risk of PCOS. Further research on this topic is needed.

Obsessive-Compulsive Symptoms in PCOS

Elsenbruch et al. (2006) found that, even after controlling for BMI, obsessive-compulsive symptomatology was higher in women with PCOS than levels typically seen in women (using normative data rather than recruiting a control group). Cesta et al. (2016) found increased risk of 'Cluster C' personality disorders in 24,385 women with PCOS, independent of other psychiatric morbidities. 'Cluster C' personality disorders include avoidant, dependent, and obsessive-compulsive personality disorder. However Cesta et al. did not analyse these three disorders separately, so we cannot say whether obsessive-compulsive personality disorder was higher in PCOS, or whether avoidant or dependent personality disorder was higher.

Autism Spectrum Disorder (ASD) and Attention Deficit Hyperactivity Disorder (ADHD)

ASD and ADHD are generally more common in boys than girls (Yang et al. 2018). Though it is possible that female autism is under-diagnosed (van Wijngaarden-Cremers 2019), generally autism is seen as four times more common in males, and Asperger syndrome (AS, the less severe version of autism), is nine times more common in males. Why is this relevant to PCOS? Well, most research points to prenatal androgenisation as being at the root of the development of PCOS (e.g. Abbott et al. 2019), and some researchers hypothesise that autism is caused by elevated prenatal androgen levels (the 'extreme male brain' theory of autism; Baron-Cohen 2002).

Initial support for the ASD/PCOS connection was provided by Ingudomnukul et al. (2007), who found that PCOS was more common in women with AS than healthy controls. However this study had an unrepresentatively low incidence of PCOS in the control group (2.7% of the 183 control women) compared to normal levels of PCOS in the Autism Spectrum Condition (ASC) group (11.3% in the 54 women with ASC). In other words, they didn't find unusually high rates of PCOS in ASD, so much as they found unusually low rates of PCOS in their control group.

Since then much more credible support for the hypothesis that PCOS and ASD/ADHD have their roots in prenatal androgenisation comes from a large GP database which found that autism and ADHD are more common in women with PCOS (Berni et al. 2018). Additional support for the PCOS/ASD link comes from Cesta et al. (2016), who found increased risk of ASD in 24,385 women with PCOS (AOR = 1.55), independent of other psychiatric morbidities. They also found a non-significantly *reduced* risk of ADHD in PCOS (AOR = 0.91).

Cognition

There appears to be no impact of PCOS on general cognitive functioning (memory, language, etc.) (Ghazeeri et al. 2013). Indeed one study has found that a specific cognitive ability related to visuo-spatial ability is increased in PCOS (Barry et al. 2013), though some other research on this might suggest that the stress and other issues associated with PCOS might interfere with cognitive performance (see 'mental rotation' in Chap. 4).

Conclusion

It appears that there is more to the psychological aspects of PCOS than anxiety and depression, and there is still a lot of work to be done in identifying and understanding these other dimensions. It is not enough to, for example, say that women with PCOS are more neurotic than other women, or that they are more at risk of autism spectrum disorder. We need to unpack these constructs and understand them in the light of the lived experiences of women with PCOS. It could be that much of what we are identifying as psychiatric risk may be explained by the body image issues of PCOS. For example, women with PCOS might be less inclined to socialise than other women due to embarrassment about their symptoms, but this behaviour could potentially be flagged as an indicator of ASD, or avoidant personality disorder. Equally, what appears to be neuroticism might be partly (or mostly?) explained by HPA problems, or hypoglycaemic episodes. At present, we are in the early data-gathering phase of research, and lot more needs to be learned before we can make more nuanced psychological assessments of women with PCOS.

References

Abbott, D. H., Dumesic, D. A., & Levine, J. E. (2019). Hyperandrogenic origins of polycystic ovary syndrome–implications for pathophysiology and therapy. *Expert Review of Endocrinology & Metabolism, 14*(2), 131–143.

Açmaz, G., Albayrak, E., Acmaz, B., Başer, M., Soyak, M., Zararsız, G., & İpekMüderris, İ. (2013). Level of anxiety, depression, self-esteem, social anxiety, and quality of life among the women with polycystic ovary syndrome. *The Scientific World Journal, 2013*, 7.

Alur-Gupta, S., Lee, I., Chemerinski, A., Chang, L., & Dokras, A. (2019). *OR25-2. Racial differences in anxiety, depression, and quality of life between white and black women with PCOS and controls.* Endo2019 abstracts. Retrieved from https://www.abstractsonline.com/pp8/#!/5752/presentation/17064.

Álvarez-Blasco, F., Luque-Ramírez, M., & Escobar-Morreale, H. F. (2010). Obesity impairs general health-related quality of life (HR-QoL) in premenopausal women to a greater extent than polycystic ovary syndrome (PCOS). *Clinical Endocrinology, 73*(5), 595–601.

American Psychiatric Association. (2013). *Diagnostic and statistical manual of mental disorders* (5th ed.). Arlington, VA: American Psychiatric Association.

Balikci, A., Erdem, M., KESKIN, U., Zincir, S. B., Guelsuen, M., Oezcelik, F., … Erguen, A. (2014). Depression, anxiety, and anger in patients with polycystic ovary syndrome. *Nöro Psikiyatri Arşivi, 51*(4), 328.

Barnard, L., Ferriday, D., Guenther, N., Strauss, B., Balen, A. H., & Dye, L. (2007). Quality of life and psychological well being in polycystic ovary syndrome. *Human Reproduction, 22*, 2279–2286.

Baron-Cohen, S. (2002). The extreme male brain theory of autism. *Trends in Cognitive Sciences, 6*(6), 248–254.

Barry, J. A., Hardiman, P. J., Saxby, B. K., & Kuczmierczyk, A. (2011a). Testosterone and mood dysfunction in women with polycystic ovarian syndrome compared to subfertile controls. *Journal of Psychosomatic Obstetrics and Gynecology, 32*(2), 104–111.

Barry, J. A., Kuczmierczyk, A. R., & Hardiman, P. J. (2011b). Anxiety and depression in polycystic ovary syndrome: A systematic review and meta-analysis. *Human Reproduction, 26*(9), 2442–2451.

Barry, J. A., Parekh, H. S. K., & Hardiman, P. J. (2013). Visual-spatial cognition in women with polycystic ovarian syndrome: The role of androgens. *Human Reproduction, 28*(10), 2832–2837.

Barry, J. A., Qu, F., & Hardiman, P. J. (2018). An exploration of the hypothesis that testosterone is implicated in the psychological functioning of women with polycystic ovary syndrome (PCOS). *Medical Hypotheses, 110*, 42–45.

Barth, J. H., Catalan, J., Cherry, C. A., & Day, A. (1993). Psychological morbidity in women referred for treatment of hirsutism. *Journal of Psychosomatic Research, 37*, 615–619.

Basirat, Z., Faramarzi, M., Esmaelzadeh, S., Mahouti, T., & Geraili, Z. (2018). Stress, depression, sexual function, and alexithymia in infertile females with and without polycystic ovary syndrome: A case-control study. *International Journal of Fertility and Sterility, 13*(3), 203–208.

Bazarganipour, F., Ziaei, S., Montazeri, A., Foroozanfard, F., Kazemnejad, A., & Faghihzadeh, S. (2013). Body image satisfaction and self-esteem status among the patients with polycystic ovary syndrome. *Iranian Journal of Reproductive Medicine, 11*(10), 829.

Benson, S., Arck, P. C., Tan, S., Hahn, S., Mann, K., Rifaie, N., … Elsenbruch, S. (2009). Disturbed stress responses in women with polycystic ovary syndrome. *Psychoneuroendocrinology, 34*(5), 727–735.

Berni, T. R., Morgan, C. L., Berni, E. R., & Rees, D. A. (2018). Polycystic ovary syndrome is associated with adverse mental health and neurodevelopmental outcomes. *The Journal of Clinical Endocrinology & Metabolism, 103*(6), 2116–2125.

Brown, P. J. (1991). Culture and the evolution of obesity. *Human Nature, 2*, 31–57.

Burger, H. G. (2002). Androgen production in women. *Fertility and Sterility, 77*, S3–S5.

Carranza-Lira, S., Velasco Díaz, G., Olivares, A., Chán Verdugo, R., & Herrera, J. (2006). Correlation of Kupperman's index with estrogen and androgen levels, according to weight and body fat distribution in postmenopausal women from Mexico City. *International Journal of Fertility and Women's Medicine, 51*, 83–88.

Cesta, C. E., Kuja-Halkola, R., Lehto, K., Iliadou, A. N., & Landén, M. (2017). Polycystic ovary syndrome, personality, and depression: A twin study. *Psychoneuroendocrinology, 85*, 63–68.

Cesta, C. E., Månsson, M., Palm, C., Lichtenstein, P., Iliadou, A. N., & Landén, M. (2016). Polycystic ovary syndrome and psychiatric disorders: Co-morbidity and heritability in a nationwide Swedish cohort. *Psychoneuroendocrinology, 73*, 196–203.

Clayton, W. J., Lipton, M., Elford, J., Rustin, M., & Sherr, L. (2005). A randomized controlled trial of laser treatment among hirsute women with polycystic ovary syndrome. *The British Journal of Dermatology, 152*, 986–992.

Coffey, S., Bano, G., & Mason, H. D. (2006). Health-related quality of life in women with polycystic ovary syndrome: A comparison with the general population using the Polycystic Ovary Syndrome Questionnaire (PCOSQ) and the Short Form-36 (SF-36). *Gynecological Endocrinology, 22*, 80–86.

Cooney, L. G., Lee, I., Sammel, M. D., & Dokras, A. (2017). High prevalence of moderate and severe depressive and anxiety symptoms in polycystic ovary syndrome: A systematic review and meta-analysis. *Human Reproduction, 32*(5), 1075–1091.

Cronin, L., Guyatt, G., Griffith, L., Wong, E., Azziz, R., Futterweit, W., … Dunaif, A. (1998). Development of a health-related quality-of-life questionnaire (PCOSQ) for women with polycystic ovary syndrome (PCOS). *The Journal of Clinical Endocrinology & Metabolism, 83*(6), 1976–1987.

De Niet, J. E., De Koning, C. M., Pastoor, H., Duivenvoorden, H. J., Valkenburg, O., Ramakers, M. J., … Laven, J. S. E. (2010). Psychological well-being and sexarche in women with polycystic ovary syndrome. *Human Reproduction, 25*(6), 1497–1503.

Deeks, A. A., Gibson-Helm, M. E., Paul, E., & Teede, H. J. (2011). Is having polycystic ovary syndrome a predictor of poor psychological function including anxiety and depression? *Human Reproduction, 26*(6), 1399–1407.

Eggers, S., & Kirchengast, S. (2001). The polycystic ovary syndrome—A medical condition but also an important psychosocial problem. *Collegium Antropologicum, 25*, 673–685.

Elsenbruch, S., Benson, S., Hahn, S., Tan, S., Mann, K., Pleger, K., … Janssen, O. E. (2006). Determinants of emotional distress in women with polycystic ovary syndrome. *Human Reproduction, 21*, 1092–1099.

Elsenbruch, S., Hahn, S., Kowalsky, D., Offner, A. H., Schedlowski, M., Mann, K., & Janssen, O. E. (2003). Quality of life, psychosocial well-being, and sexual satisfaction in women with polycystic ovary syndrome. *The Journal of Clinical Endocrinology and Metabolism, 88*, 5801–5807.

Emeksiz, H. C., Bideci, A., Nalbantoğlu, B., Nalbantoğlu, A., Celik, C., Yulaf, Y., … Cinaz, P. (2018). Anxiety and depression states of adolescents with polycystic ovary syndrome. *Turkish Journal of Medical Sciences, 48*(3), 531–536.

Eysenck, H. J., & Eysenck, M. W. (1987). *Personality and individual differences.* New York: Plenum.

Faith, M. S., Flint, J., Fairburn, C. G., Goodwin, G. M., & Allison, D. B. (2001). Gender differences in the relationship between personality dimensions and relative body weight. *Obesity Research, 9*, 647–650.

Farrell, K., & Antoni, M. H. (2010). Insulin resistance, obesity, inflammation, and depression in polycystic ovary syndrome: Biobehavioral mechanisms and interventions. *Fertility and Sterility, 94*(5), 1565–1574.

Fernandez, R. C., Moore, V. M., Van Ryswyk, E. M., Varcoe, T. J., Rodgers, R. J., March, W. A., … Davies, M. J. (2018). Sleep disturbances in women with polycystic ovary syndrome: Prevalence, pathophysiology, impact and management strategies. *Nature and Science of Sleep, 10*, 45.

Fogel, R. B., Malhotra, A., Pillar, G., Pittman, S. D., Dunaif, A., & White, D. P. (2001). Increased prevalence of obstructive sleep apnea syndrome in obese women with polycystic ovary syndrome. *The Journal of Clinical Endocrinology and Metabolism, 86*(3), 1175–1180.

Franik, G., Krysta, K., Madej, P., Gimlewicz-Pięta, B., Oślizło, B., Trukawka, J., & Olszanecka-Glinianowicz, M. (2016). Sleep disturbances in women with polycystic ovary syndrome. *Gynecological Endocrinology, 32*(12), 1014–1017.

Gallinelli, A., Matteo, M. L., Volpe, A., & Facchinetti, F. (2000). Autonomic and neuroendocrine responses to stress in patients with functional hypothalamic secondary amenorrhea. *Fertility and Sterility, 73*(4), 812–816.

Ghazeeri, G., Fakih, A., Abbas, H. A., Harajly, S., & Awwad, J. (2013). Anxiety, cognitive, and depressive assessment in adolescents with polycystic ovarian syndrome: A pilot study. *Journal of Pediatric and Adolescent Gynecology, 26*(5), 269–273.

Goyal, M., & Dawood, A. S. (2017). Debates regarding lean patients with polycystic ovary syndrome: A narrative review. *Journal of Human Reproductive Sciences, 10*(3), 154.

Greenwood, E. A., Pasch, L. A., Cedars, M. I., Legro, R. S., Huddleston, H. G., & Network, H. D. R. M., & Eunice Kennedy Shriver National Institute of Child Health. (2018). Association among depression, symptom experience, and quality of life in polycystic ovary syndrome. *American Journal of Obstetrics and Gynecology, 219*(3), 279–e1.

Greiner, M., Paredes, A., Araya, V., & Lara, H. E. (2005). Role of stress and sympathetic innervation in the development of polycystic ovary syndrome. *Endocrine, 28*(3), 319–324.

Guyatt, G., Weaver, B., Cronin, L., Dooley, J. A., & Azziz, R. (2004). Health related quality of life in PCOS. *Journal of Clinical Epidemiology, 57,* 1279–1287.

Hahn, S., Benson, S., Elsenbruch, S., Pleger, K., Tan, S., Mann, K., … Janssen, O. E. (2006). Metformin treatment of polycystic ovary syndrome improves health-related quality-of-life, emotional distress and sexuality. *Human Reproduction, 21,* 1925–1934.

Hettema, J. M., Prescott, C. A., & Kendler, K. S. (2004). Genetic and environmental sources of covariation between generalized anxiety disorder and neuroticism. *American Journal of Psychiatry, 161*(9), 1581–1587.

Himelein, M. J., & Thatcher, S. S. (2006a). Depression and body image among women with polycystic ovary syndrome. *Journal of Health Psychology, 11*(4), 613–625.

Himelein, M. J., & Thatcher, S. S. (2006b). Polycystic ovary syndrome and mental health: A review. *Obstetrical & Gynecological Survey, 61*(11), 723–732.

Hung, J. H., Hu, L. Y., Tsai, S. J., Yang, A. C., Huang, M. W., Chen, P. M., … Shen, C. C. (2014). Risk of psychiatric disorders following polycystic ovary syndrome: A nationwide population-based cohort study. *PLoS One, 9*(5), e97041.

Ingudomnukul, E., Baron-Cohen, S., Wheelwright, S., & Knickmeyer, R. (2007). Elevated rates of testosterone-related disorders in women with autism spectrum conditions. *Hormones and Behavior, 51*, 597–604.

Jones, G. L., Benes, K., Clark, T. L., Denham, R., Holder, M. G., Haynes, T. J., … Balen, A. (2004). The polycystic ovary syndrome health-related quality of life questionnaire (PCOSQ): A validation. *Human Reproduction, 19*(2), 371–377.

Jones, G. L., Hall, J. M., Balen, A. H., & Ledger, W. L. (2007). Health-related quality of life measurement in women with polycystic ovary syndrome: A systematic review. *Human Reproduction Update, 14*(1), 15–25.

Kahal, H., Kyrou, I., Tahrani, A. A., & Randeva, H. S. (2017). Obstructive sleep apnoea and polycystic ovary syndrome: A comprehensive review of clinical interactions and underlying pathophysiology. *Clinical Endocrinology, 87*(4), 313–319.

Karimah, P., & Hestiantoro, A. (2016). The cut off of Ferriman Gallwey Score for PCOS in Asia and the degree of hyperandrogenism indicator. *KnE Medicine*, 186–192. https://doi.org/10.18502/kme.v1i1.640.

Kawamura, S., Maesawa, C., Nakamura, K., Nakayama, K., Morita, M., Hiruma, Y., … Masuda, T. (2011). Predisposition for borderline personality disorder with comorbid major depression is associated with that for polycystic ovary syndrome in female Japanese population. *Neuropsychiatric Disease and Treatment, 7*, 655.

Keegan, A., Liao, L. M., & Boyle, M. (2003). 'Hirsutism': A psychological analysis. *Journal of Health Psychology, 8*(3), 327–345.

Kitzinger, C., & Willmott, J. (2002). The thief of womanhood': Women's experience of polycystic ovarian syndrome. *Social Science & Medicine, 54*, 349–361.

Klipstein, K. G., & Goldberg, J. F. (2006). Screening for bipolar disorder in women with polycystic ovary syndrome. *Journal of Affective Disorders, 91*(2–3), 205–209.

Kolotkin, R. L., Meter, K., & Williams, G. R. (2001). Quality of life and obesity. *Obesity Reviews, 2*, 219–229.

Kumarapeli, V., Seneviratne, R. D. A., Wijeyaratne, C. N., Yapa, R. M. S. C., & Dodampahala, S. H. (2008). A simple screening approach for assessing community prevalence and phenotype of polycystic ovary syndrome in a semiurban population in Sri Lanka. *American Journal of Epidemiology, 168*(3), 321–328.

Legro, R. S., Schlaff, W. D., Diamond, M. P., Coutifaris, C., Casson, P. R., Brzyski, R. G., … Ohl, D. (2010). Total testosterone assays in women with polycystic ovary syndrome: Precision and correlation with hirsutism. *The Journal of Clinical Endocrinology & Metabolism, 95*(12), 5305–5313.

Lin, T. Y., Lin, P. Y., Su, T. P., Li, C. T., Lin, W. C., Chang, W. H., … Chen, M. H. (2017). Risk of developing obstructive sleep apnea among women with polycystic ovarian syndrome: A nationwide longitudinal follow-up study. *Sleep Medicine, 36*, 165–169.

Lipton, M. G., Sherr, L., Elford, J., Rustin, M. H., & Clayton, W. J. (2006). Women living with facial hair: The psychological and behavioral burden. *Journal of Psychosomatic Research, 61*, 161–168.

Mącik, D. (2016). Loss of attributes of femininity, anxiety and value crisis. Women with polycystic ovary syndrome compared to women after mastectomy and in menopause. *Health Psychology Report, 4*(2), 159–169.

Manlove, H. A., Guillermo, C., & Gray, P. B. (2008). Do women with polycystic ovary syndrome (PCOS) report differences in sex-typed behavior as children and adolescents?: Results of a pilot study. *Annals of Human Biology, 35*, 584–595.

Månsson, M., Holte, J., Landin-Wilhelmsen, K., Dahlgren, E., Johansson, A., & Landén, M. (2008). Women with polycystic ovary syndrome are often depressed or anxious—A case control study. *Psychoneuroendocrinology, 33*, 1132–1138.

Mayo Clinic. (2019). Personality disorders. Retrieved May 7, 2019, from https://www.mayoclinic.org/diseases-conditions/personality-disorders/symptoms-causes/syc-20354463.

McCook, J. G. (2002). *The influence of hyperandrogenism, obesity and infertility on the psychosocial health and well-being of women with polycystic ovary syndrome*. Unpublished doctoral dissertation, University of Michigan, Ann Arbor, MI.

McCook, J. G., Reame, N. E., & Thatcher, S. S. (2005). Health-related quality of life issues in women with polycystic ovary syndrome. *Journal of Obstetric, Gynecologic, and Neonatal Nursing, 34*, 12–20.

Modell, E., Goldstein, D., & Reyes, F. I. (1990). Endocrine and behavioral responses to psychological stress in hyperandrogenic women. *Fertility and Sterility, 53*(3), 454–459.

Moghadam, Z. B., Fereidooni, B., Saffari, M., & Montazeri, A. (2018). Measures of health-related quality of life in PCOS women: A systematic review. *International Journal of Women's Health, 10*, 397.

Monzani, F., Pucci, F., Caraccio, N., Bagnolesi, A., Molli, D., Fenu, A., & Prunetti, C. (1994). Psychological and psychopathological correlates in the polycystic ovary syndrome (PCOS). *Medicina–Psicosomatica, 39*, 225–236.

Moran, L. J., March, W. A., Whitrow, M. J., Giles, L. C., Davies, M. J., & Moore, V. M. (2015). Sleep disturbances in a community-based sample of women with polycystic ovary syndrome. *Human Reproduction, 30*(2), 466–472.

Moss, M. (2016, April 19). PCOS: Causes, symptoms and treatment for PCOS. *Huffington Post*. Retrieved from https://www.huffingtonpost.co.uk/entry/pcos-causes-symptoms-and-treatment_uk_570e7347e4b01711c612daaa?ncid=engmodushpmg00000004&guccounter=1&guce_referrer_us=aHR0cHM6Ly90LmNvL0FXd2NtOXhhaWWs&guce_referrer_cs=RNBbOvg7nX04gTsRS6AoSw.

Nelson-DeGrave, V. L., Wickenheisser, J. K., Cockrell, J. E., Wood, J. R., Legro, R. S., Strauss, J. F., & McAllister, J. M. (2004). Valproate potentiates androgen biosynthesis in human ovarian theca cells. *Endocrinology, 145*, 799–808.

Palomba, S., Giallauria, F., Falbo, A., Russo, T., Oppedisano, R., Tolino, A., … Orio, F. (2007). Structured exercise training programme versus hypocaloric hyperproteic diet in obese polycystic ovary syndrome patients with anovulatory infertility: A 24-week pilot study. *Human Reproduction, 23*(3), 642–650.

Pastore, L. M., Patrie, J. T., Morris, W. L., Dalal, P., & Bray, M. J. (2011). Depression symptoms and body dissatisfaction association among polycystic ovary syndrome women. *Journal of Psychosomatic Research, 71*(4), 270–276.

Pervin, L. A. (1994). A critical analysis of current trait theory. *Psychological Inquiry, 5*(2), 103–113.

Pfister, G., & Rømer, K. (2017). "It's not very feminine to have a mustache": Experiences of Danish women with polycystic ovary syndrome. *Health Care for Women International, 38*(2), 167–186.

Rasgon, N. L., Altshuler, L. L., Fairbanks, L., Elman, S., Bitran, J., Labarca, R., … Suppes, T. (2005). Reproductive function and risk for PCOS in women treated for bipolar disorder. *Bipolar Disorders, 7*, 246–259.

Reiche, E. M. V., Nunes, S. O. V., & Morimoto, H. K. (2004). Stress, depression, the immune system, and cancer. *The Lancet Oncology, 5*(10), 617–625.

Sahingöz, M., Uguz, F., Gezginc, K., & Korucu, D. G. (2013). Axis I and Axis II diagnoses in women with PCOS. *General Hospital Psychiatry, 35*(5), 508–511.

Scaruffi, E., Gambineri, A., Cattaneo, S., Turra, J., Vettor, R., & Mioni, R. (2014). Personality and psychiatric disorders in women affected by polycystic ovary syndrome. *Frontiers in Endocrinology, 5,* 185.

Shipley, B. A., Weiss, A., Der, G., Taylor, M. D., & Deary, I. J. (2007). Neuroticism, extraversion, and mortality in the UK Health and Lifestyle Survey: A 21-year prospective cohort study. *Psychosomatic Medicine, 69,* 923–931.

Sonino, N., Fava, G. A., Mani, E., Belluardo, P., & Boscaro, M. (1993). Quality of life of hirsute women. *Postgraduate Medical Journal, 69,* 186–189.

Spielberger, C. D., Sydeman, S. J., Owen, A. E., & Marsh, B. J. (1999). Measuring anxiety and anger with the State-Trait Anxiety Inventory (STAI) and the State-Trait Anger Expression Inventory (STAXI). In M. E. Maruish (Ed.), *The use of psychological testing for treatment planning and outcomes assessment* (pp. 993–1021). Mahwah, NJ: Lawrence Erlbaum Associates Publishers.

Stellman, S. D., Takezaki, T., Wang, L., Chen, Y., Citron, M. L., Djordjevic, M. V., … Ogawa, H. (2001). Smoking and lung cancer risk in American and Japanese men: An international case-control study. *Cancer Epidemiology and Prevention Biomarkers, 10*(11), 1193–1199.

Suri, J., Suri, J. C., Chatterjee, B., Mittal, P., & Adhikari, T. (2016). Obesity may be the common pathway for sleep-disordered breathing in women with polycystic ovary syndrome. *Sleep Medicine, 23,* 32–39.

Tasali, E., Van Cauter, E., & Ehrmann, D. A. (2006). Relationships between sleep disordered breathing and glucose metabolism in polycystic ovary syndrome. *The Journal of Clinical Endocrinology and Metabolism, 91*(1), 36–42.

Tasali, E., Van Cauter, E., Hoffman, L., & Ehrmann, D. A. (2008). Impact of obstructive sleep apnea on insulin resistance and glucose tolerance in women with polycystic ovary syndrome. *The Journal of Clinical Endocrinology and Metabolism, 93*(10), 3878–3884.

Trent, M. E., Rich, M., Austin, S. B., & Gordon, C. M. (2002). Quality of life in adolescent girls with polycystic ovary syndrome. *Archives of Pediatrics & Adolescent Medicine, 156*(6), 556–560.

Trent, M., Austin, S. B., Rich, M., & Gordon, C. M. (2005). Overweight status of adolescent girls with polycystic ovary syndrome: Body mass index as mediator of quality of life. *Ambulatory Pediatrics, 5,* 107–111.

Verhaak, C. M., Smeenk, J. M., van Minnen, A., Kremer, J. A., & Kraaimaat, F. W. (2005). A longitudinal, prospective study on emotional adjustment before, during and after consecutive fertility treatment cycles. *Human Reproduction, 20,* 2253–2260.

Wake, D. J., Strand, M., Rask, E., Westerbacka, J., Livingstone, D. E., Soderberg, S., … Walker, B. R. (2007). Intra-adipose sex steroid metabolism and body fat distribution in idiopathic human obesity. *Clinical Endocrinology, 66*, 440–446.

van Wijngaarden-Cremers, P. (2019). Autism in boys and girls, women and men throughout the lifespan. In J. A. Barry, R. Kingerlee, M. J. Seager, & L. Sullivan (Eds.), *The Palgrave Handbook of Male Psychology and Mental Health*. London: Palgrave Macmillan.

Ware, J. E., Jr., & Sherbourne, C. D. (1992). The MOS 36-item short-form health survey (SF-36): I. conceptual framework and item selection. *Medical Care, 30*, 473–483.

Williams, S., Sheffield, D., & Knibb, R. C. (2018). The polycystic ovary syndrome quality of life scale (PCOSQOL): Development and preliminary validation. *Health Psychology Open, 5*(2), 2055102918788195.

Xie, J., Bi, Q., Shang, W., Yan, M., Yang, Y., Miao, D., & Zhang, H. (2012). Positive and negative relationship between anxiety and depression of patients in pain: A bifactor model analysis. *PLoS One, 7*(10), e47577.

Yang, E. Y., Lee, D. K., & Yang, J. H. (2018). Environmental endocrine disruptors and neurological disorders. *Journal of the Korean Neurological Association, 36*(3), 139–144.

Zigmond, A. S., & Snaith, R. P. (1983). The hospital anxiety and depression scale. *Acta Psychiatrica Scandinavica, 67*(6), 361–370.

4

Impact of Testosterone on Aspects of Psychology

Abstract This chapter explores what we know about the psychological effects of testosterone in women, both with polycystic ovary syndrome (PCOS) and without. Many readers will find this chapter fascinating. The topics include ones that people might think they know about, but are widely misunderstood, such as sexual orientation and aggression. There are other topics in which testosterone has the expected impact on healthy women (such as cognition and libido), but works differently in women with PCOS. There are many surprises in this chapter, not least the evidence that testosterone, a prosocial hormone.

Keywords Mental rotation • Libido • Sexual orientation • Aggression • Prosocial

This chapter will explore some of the evidence of a relationship between testosterone (and other androgens) and psychology. Many people find this subject fascinating, probably because it speaks to the intuitive sense of the power of hormones. Testosterone is not only a sex hormone, but 'the male hormone', one which can increase or decrease the physical characteristics of masculinity. However, there are some enduring myths and misunderstandings about testosterone. It's true that too much testosterone is unhealthy for women (and too little is unhealthy for men), but we often forget that the right amount of testosterone is key to the health of women and men.

As noted in Chap. 1, ovarian androgen receptors are key to healthy ovulation (Astapova et al. 2019), and in many ways the healthy balance of testosterone to estrogen is what is important. However, such nuances are often lost these days in the popular narrative of testosterone as the hormone of violence (Dunphy 2018) and mental health problems (e.g. autism). Some have even used the pejorative term 'testosterone poisoning' to explain macho behaviour (Booth et al. 2006).

Testosterone Levels in PCOS

Although testosterone is one of the key features of polycystic ovary syndrome (PCOS), we know from the Rotterdam criteria (Chap. 1) that it is not necessary for a diagnosis of PCOS. On the other hand, if a PCOS diagnosis is made without reference to testosterone, then polycystic ovaries are present and this indicates that the ovaries are producing testosterone. In fact, around 30% of women with PCOS show elevated testosterone levels (Azziz et al. 2009). But what are the levels of testosterone seen in PCOS? The answer is complex, because levels vary due to a range of factors, including the type of assay method (see below) and the laboratory equipment used. Using the most accurate assay method (mass spectrometry), 188 women with PCOS had mean (SD) testosterone levels (in nmol/L) of 1.43 (1.35–1.45), compared to 1.11 (1.04–1.17) in 202 control women (Schüring et al. 2016). Using a basic assay method (a chemiluminescence immunoassay) with the same women found similar results: PCOS 1.48 (1.40–1.71), controls 1.00 (0.91–1.08). In other words, we could say that, taking the most accurate assay method, testosterone levels are roughly a third higher in PCOS than in healthy women.

As you can see, only relatively small elevations from the norm are needed to cause an imbalance. In contrast, very high levels of androgens are seen prenatally in congenital adrenal hyperplasia (CAH), which are probably similar to the levels seen in a healthy male fetus at around week 13 of gestation, which are in turn similar to the levels seen in boys going through puberty.

Care should be taken when reading the laboratory results of assays, because various different units of measurement are commonly used, depending on the country and the laboratory. In PCOS research today, units are most often expressed in ng/mL, or else nmol/L. The testosterone values appear to vary widely depending on the units used, and a conversion table can be very useful (see Table S4 in Barry et al. 2011b).

There are various ways of measuring ('assaying') testosterone (for a simple description, see Barry et al. 2011b). The most accurate is liquid chromatography mass spectrometry, but this is rarely used in routine clinical work. The most commonly used method is direct radioimmunoassay (RIA), but this is relatively inaccurate in terms of measuring testosterone because it cross-reacts with other biochemicals such as 11-keto-testosterone, 11-beta-OH-testosterone, and dihydrotestosterone (Roche Diagnostics 2000). This makes RIA a more general measure of the presence of androgens, which arguably could make it a better measure if your aim is to find out about the impact of androgens in general rather than testosterone in particular. Legro et al. (2010) found that results from the two methods (RIA and tandem mass spectrometry) correlate reasonably well, making the accuracy of methods a matter of how much you want to measure testosterone in particular, and how much you want to measure androgens in general (or androgenic potential). But for accurately measuring testosterone in the low levels typically seen in women, the best advice is from Rosner et al. (2007) who recommend liquid chromatography mass spectrometry.

Similar to the issue of measuring androgenic potential versus testosterone, it is also considered better to measure 'free' testosterone, that is, testosterone that has not been made inert by being bound to SHBG (sex hormone binding globulin). Taking SHBG into account is useful because if testosterone levels are high, but SHBG levels are also high, then the biological impact of testosterone on PCOS symptoms is likely to be low. When SHBG is taken into account, the measure of testosterone is called 'free testosterone', expressed as the free testosterone index (FTI) or more commonly the free androgen index (FAI). Thus, free testosterone is a better measure for PCOS, though it is not always used in clinical practice or research.

When the term 'testosterone' is used in this book, I am usually referring to total testosterone, typically measured using a method other than tandem mass spectrometry. This reflects the fact that more sophisticated methods of analysis have become available only in recent years, and guidelines issued only in the past decade or so; thus, much of the research on PCOS has tended to use the more basic methods. This puts a question mark over some of the findings of research cited in this book: was testosterone measured, or androgens? Was an effect of testosterone overlooked because the assay method was not sensitive enough? Although future research should use appropriate measures and guidelines, we should not be unduly dismissive of existing research using measures and techniques which have made valuable discoveries and form a good basis for further research.

Another measurement issue to be aware of is that in healthy women, testosterone levels vary throughout the day (lowest in the early evening), by month (lowest during menstruation), and over the lifespan (gradually getting lower from the late 30s). It is recommended that in healthy women the timing of taking blood samples is standardised, and are taken in the morning and in the first few days of the menstrual cycle (early follicular phase) (Davis 2001).

Testosterone and Cognition

The impact of testosterone on cognition is interesting, because there is lots of research suggesting that people with more testosterone tend to do better on a particular cognitive task—3-D mental rotation. This task involves being able to imagine what an object looks like from various perspectives. The classic test is the Shepard-Metzler 'cubes' (Shepard and Metzler 1971), where participants are rated on their ability to imagine irregular objects rotated in space. Men tend to do better than women on this task, and two studies have found that administering testosterone to women helps them to do better on tasks involving spatial abilities (Aleman et al. 2004; Pintzka et al. 2016).

The evidence for the impact of testosterone on cognition in PCOS is mixed, probably due to methodological differences between studies. It seems likely that the effect is mostly specific to mental rotation tasks in particular rather than visuo-spatial tasks in general. Barry et al. (2013) found, in a study of 69 women with PCOS and 41 subfertile controls, that testosterone was significantly positively correlated with 3-D mental rotation scores, whereas estradiol was significantly negatively correlated with 3-D mental rotation scores. These correlations were seen in the PCOS group only. Significantly higher scores on the mental rotation task were seen only in the 19 hyperandrogenic PCOS women (with testosterone levels >2.9 nmol/L).

There is a lot of evidence showing that testosterone is related to better 3-D mental rotation ability in non-PCOS populations (see Barry and Owens 2019), making this ability one of the few positive points for women with PCOS. Three other studies of PCOS and mental rotation scoring have not found the effect seen in Barry et al., probably due to methodological limitations. Schattmann and Sherwin (2007) had a small sample (22 PCOS and 22 controls), used a bespoke diagnosis of PCOS (a variation of the National Institutes of Health (NIH) criteria), and gave participants longer to complete the task than prescribed by Peters et al. (1995), which would disadvantage those who are naturally faster at the task. Barnard et al. (2007) had a large sample (135 PCOS and 322 healthy controls) but, like Schattmann and Sherwin, also deviated from the protocol of Peters et al., this time by presenting participants with one instead of four alternative figures. Furthermore, being an internet-based study, they couldn't measure testosterone, which is a key variable of interest in this research. Udiawar (2017) did not find improved mental rotation in PCOS, probably because a mental rotation task as such was not used—the Rey-Osterrieth Complex Figure Test (ROCF) was used instead.

But perhaps there is a more obvious reason why some research hasn't found that women with PCOS score higher on mental rotation tasks. An interesting study by Lujan and Mergler (2015) found that 79 women with PCOS scored significantly *worse* than 40 healthy women on tests of spatial ability, including on the mental rotation task. Testosterone was not related to scoring, but menstrual cycle length, number of follicles per ovary, and triglycerides (fat levels in the bloodstream) were each independent predictors of mental rotation scoring in the PCOS group. The authors suggest that these variables indicate that reproductive and metabolic abnormalities may have reduced task performance in PCOS. Based on these findings we might speculate that the effect of testosterone, normally the key biochemical facilitating 3-D mental rotation, may be eclipsed in PCOS by the various problems of PCOS, which—ironically—are caused by testosterone. We saw in Chap. 3 studies where the HPA reactivity of women with PCOS caused heightened stress when doing simple cognitive tasks (Modell et al. 1990; Gallinelli et al. 2000), and it is well recognised that stress can interfere with performance on tasks, so it could be that in PCOS heightened anxiety and other phenomena seen in PCOS (e.g. sleepiness from sleep apnoea, or confusion caused by hypoglycaemia—see Chap. 5) might conspire against scoring on this task.

Testosterone and Libido

So far in this book we have mainly been discussing the problem for women of having too much testosterone, so it might be surprising to know that there are problems for women of having too little testosterone. Typically the psychological symptoms associated with this are loss of sexual desire, lower mood and feeling of tiredness, decreased assertiveness, and reduced confidence (Davis 2001). If the lack of testosterone endures, there are long-term implications for bone mass and muscle strength.

Most of what is known about testosterone and libido comes from non-PCOS women. Although there is no sharp decline in testosterone in women as happens with estrogen in menopause, levels drop steadily from as early as the late 30s. As well as diminishing libido, it can diminish general intimacy, passion, and mood (Davis 2001). Nathorst-Böös et al. (2006) conducted a randomised control trial (RCT) with 77 postmenopausal women on hormone replacement therapy (HRT). They were randomised to receive either 10 mg testosterone gel or placebo control over three months. The testosterone had positive effects on various aspects of sexual life, including frequency of sexual fantasies, arousal, activity, and orgasm. Although there was a significant increase in anxiety in the testosterone group compared to controls ($p < 0.001$), this reduced over three months ($p < 0.03$) despite the accumulation of circulating testosterone, and there was no increase in depression over the study period. Moreover, there was an overall significant increase in the Psychological General Well-Being (PGWB) scale, particularly in vitality ($p < 0.005$).

There is plenty of evidence that testosterone replacement therapy is effective in improving all of the symptoms of androgen deficiency in women (e.g. Taher et al. 2008) though there is no agreed-upon definition of androgen deficiency in women, which makes diagnosis difficult (Davis 2001).

In PCOS, however, the evidence regarding the impact of testosterone on libido is mixed, and sometimes even shows the opposite pattern (Rellini et al. 2013; Ercan et al. 2013; see also Chap. 6), possibly because testosterone is at levels high enough to cause issues that impact a woman's sense of attractiveness. If this is the case, it is similar to the effect of testosterone on 3-D mental rotation proposed above—the side effects outweigh the benefits at higher levels of testosterone.

Testosterone and Sexual Orientation

The relationship between PCOS and sexuality is inevitably a controversial topic. Sexuality is in many ways a private matter, and asking people about their sexuality doesn't always get you a clear or accurate answer, partly because of embarrassment, but also sometimes due to identity. For example, you are likely to find a greater number of people saying they have non-heterosexual attraction or experience than saying they identify as bisexual or gay. This is what Smith et al. (2003) found in their survey in Australia of 9134 women, which found that 2.2% identified as lesbian or bisexual, but 15.1% reported some degree of same-sex attraction or experience. We should expect that all studies on topics that people might feel are private or embarrassing will be prone to 'social desirability bias', and might underestimate the variable being measured.

The topic of gender and sexual orientation is relevant to PCOS because of the theory that PCOS is caused by elevated prenatal androgen, and the knowledge that in congenital adrenal hyperplasia (CAH)—which is caused by high levels of prenatal androgens—there can be an effect on sexuality. Even when such cases are treated early in life (genitalia are surgically feminised, hormone therapy is given, and they are raised as completely normal girls) women with CAH are more likely to be bisexual or lesbian. For example, Dittman et al. (1992) found that 44% of females with CAH, compared to 0% of their unaffected sisters, either desired or had experienced sexual relations with women. This is interesting evidence, but the fact that the rate of atypical sexuality is not 100% in women with CAH indicates that prenatal exposure to androgen does not fully account for sexual orientation. Also it should be noted that surgical correction of ambiguous genitalia does not always create genitals identical to most women's, and this may account for the reduced sexual interest and activity sometimes found in women with CAH (Zucker et al. 1996).

A few studies have found some evidence, though not conclusive, that PCOS is more common in female-to-male transsexuals. Futterweit et al. (1986) found an increased rate of PCOS in 40 female-to-male transsexuals. Balen et al. (1993) found that 93% of 16 female-to-male transsexuals, with no history of hormone treatment, had polycystic ovaries (not the syndrome). This is a high rate, though it should be noted that polycystic ovaries (not the syndrome) are fairly common, and may exist in around a quarter or more women who don't have PCOS. Bosinski et al. (1997) found a higher rate of polycystic ovaries in eight out of nine female-to-male (FTM) transsexuals, but did not scan fifteen healthy control women, and they estimated—based on hormonal and clinical criteria—that around two-thirds of FTM transsexuals had PCOS compared to 7% of control women. In the largest study of PCOS and FTM transsexuals, a study in Japan found that, prior to hormone treatment or surgery, of the 69 FTM cases, 40 (58.0%) had PCOS (Baba et al. 2006). Although sample sizes are mostly small given that FTM transsexualism is not particularly common, the small sample sizes and small number of studies (spanning three decades) indicates that the evidence of a connection between PCOS and transsexualism is not particularly strong. We might also speculate about file-drawer effects in this topic (the phenomenon where studies that don't have interesting findings don't get put forward for publication, or don't get published).

There is some research evidence, though again not well replicated, that being overweight, having polycystic ovaries or PCOS, and having elevated testosterone are associated with lesbianism. Boehmer et al. (2007) found that lesbian women were roughly twice as likely to be overweight as heterosexual women. In a study of 254 lesbian women and 364 heterosexual women, Agrawal et al. (2004) found a significantly higher prevalence of PCOS in lesbian women (38% vs 14%), and significantly higher androgen concentrations in lesbian women compared with heterosexual women. There was also a greater prevalence of polycystic ovaries in lesbian women (80% vs 32%).

In contrast to the findings of Agrawal et al. (2004), de Sutter et al. (2008) found that of 174 lesbian women and 200 heterosexual women attending a fertility clinic, PCOS was no more likely to be diagnosed in lesbian women (8% had PCOS) than heterosexual women (8.7% had PCOS). Manlove et al. (2008) found a greater number of women with PCOS identified as being bisexual compared to controls, but this trend was non-significant (perhaps due to the small sample size); 4 of 34 women (11%) of the PCOS group were bisexual compared to 0 of 27 controls. Nordqvist et al. (2014) found similar rates of PCOS in 124 heterosexual women (7.2%) and 171 lesbian women (7.3%).

Why has the finding of Agrawal et al. (2004) not been replicated? Well, it could be their results don't generalise to most women with PCOS because the women in the Agrawal et al. study were not really representative of the average woman with PCOS (technically called 'sample bias'). The Agrawal et al. sample might be unusual because they were recruited from a private clinic at a time when IVF was not freely available on the National Health Service (NHS) to lesbian couples. Thus, this clinic attracted a relatively high number of lesbian couples with fertility problems, and because PCOS is one of the most common fertility problems, and lesbian couples couldn't get fertility treatment paid for at NHS clinics, it is understandable that they found an unusually high number of lesbians with PCOS at their clinic. So although the findings of Agrawal et al. would generalise well to the women their clinic attracted at the time, they don't generalise very well to the average woman with PCOS. It should be noted that Agrawal et al. did not say 'Most lesbians have

PCOS, therefore most women with PCOS are lesbians', though some people made this interpretation.

Another potential weakness of the Agrawal et al. (2004) study was that the researchers were not blind to sexual orientation, which may have influenced the findings in unknown, perhaps unconscious, ways. In a study blind to the patient's sexual orientation, Smith et al. (2011) found no significant difference between the rates of PCOS in 114 lesbian and 97 heterosexual women with PCOS (7.9% and 4.1%, respectively). Some PCOS-related factors were found slightly higher in lesbian compared to heterosexual women; these did not reach statistical significance: polycystic ovaries (10.5% vs 6.2%), hirsutism (24.6% vs 15.5%), oligomenorrhea (3.6% vs 5.4%), acne in adulthood (21.1% vs 24.7%), testosterone (1.69 ng/mL vs 1.52 ng/mL), and androstenedione (1.63 ng/mL vs 1.51).

Some other studies have found partial evidence for a relationship between PCOS and sexual orientation, but, taken together, the evidence is not strong. For example, in a study of Taiwanese women, the only differences between 8 lesbians with PCOS and 89 heterosexual women with PCOS was that lesbian women had higher BMI than the others (26.5 ± 1.9 vs 22.5 ± 0.55; $p < 0.05$) (Chen et al. 2014). No doubt people will continue to find this topic of interest, but in the light of subsequent evidence from Cesta et al. (2016), we have to conclude that the weight of evidence is not in favour of an effect of PCOS on sexuality or gender. Cesta et al. found no difference between 24,385 women with PCOS and control women on gender identity disorders (AOR = 1.47) or transsexualism (AOR = 1.26), independent of psychiatric morbidities.

In their review of studies of sexual orientation in gynaecological conditions, Robinson et al. concluded regarding PCOS: 'existing notions about PCOS must be undone, and clinicians should not treat sexuality as an association' (Robinson et al. 2017, p. 390). Therefore, in contrast to some interpretations of Agrawal et al. (2004), lesbians are unlikely to be significantly more likely to have PCOS than are heterosexual women, and women with PCOS are not significantly more likely to be lesbians.

Testosterone and Aggression in PCOS and Healthy People

It is 'common knowledge' that testosterone causes aggression. So wide-spread is this notion that it has even been used as mitigating circumstances in a court case where a woman with PCOS had charges of domestic violence dropped against her because she blamed her behaviour on her 'male hormones' (Dunphy 2018). So what is the evidence that testosterone causes aggression in PCOS?

In one of the first studies of the psychological aspects of PCOS, Monzani et al. (1994) found that compared to 20 age-matched healthy controls, 23 women with PCOS showed elevations (though non-significant) on Type A personality, a personality type associated with dominance, time urgency, hostility, competitiveness/leadership, and coronary heart disease (CHD). Although they did not measure testosterone, the underlying assumption is that elevations in ratings related to dominance and aggression were caused by the elevated testosterone often seen in PCOS. However, this is an assumption rather than a fact, and is sometimes invoked without appropriate evidence being presented. For example, Gul et al. (2018) studied 28 adolescents with PCOS and 16 healthy adolescents matched on age and BMI. The PCOS group was newly diagnosed with PCOS at a hospital clinic and the controls were recruited from the same hospital but for respiratory infections. Using the State-Trait Anger Expression Inventory (STAXI) and State-Trait Anxiety Inventory (STAI) they found that the PCOS group scored higher than the control group on two subscales of anger (externalised anger $p < 0.011$; internalised anger $p < 0.08$) and two subscales of anxiety (state $p < 0.003$; trait $p < 0.0001$) and lower on anger control ($p < 0.0001$). They also found that, in the PCOS group only, anxiety was negatively associated with anger control (i.e. those with less anxiety were less likely to control their anger). Although testosterone was measured in the PCOS group, the authors did not report any test of correlation between testosterone and anger despite correlating each of the anger and anxiety subscales. This seems a lost opportunity to test for an association between testosterone and aggression, and the authors' conclusion that hyperandrogenemia might explain the findings is unsubstantiated by their findings. In another Turkish study, Balikci et al. (2014) compared 44 women with PCOS to healthy women matched on BMI. They found significantly higher levels of traits such as anger, anger-out, anger-in, and anxiety and depression, and significantly lower anger control, in the PCOS group. Again, like in the Gul et al. case, although testosterone was measured in the PCOS group, the authors did not report any test of correlation between testosterone and anger despite correlating other hormones with psychological outcomes. Barry et al. (2011a) assessed 76 women with PCOS and 49 subfertile control women on measures of anxiety, depression, and aggression levels. Testosterone levels were also tested for any relationship with the psychological outcomes. Variables that might impact the psychological measures were controlled either by study design (fertility status was similar in both groups) or statistically (age and BMI were covariates in multivariate analysis of covariance (MANCOVA)). The PCOS group was found to have significantly higher depression, anxiety, and worse quality of life (QoL) scores (apart from QoL for fertility), was significantly more neurotic (see Chap. 3 for a description of neuroticism), and scored significantly higher on two measures of anger (anger symptoms and withholding feelings of anger). However, correlations with testosterone did not explain the mood states. The pattern of findings in the three studies are interestingly similar—higher anger expression, higher withheld anger, and higher anxiety, though these findings cannot be explained as being a consequence of elevated testosterone.

Several studies of women with PCOS have either not found a link between testosterone and depression (Hahn et al. 2005; McCook 2002; Rasgon et al. 2003) or had weak or mixed findings. An interesting example of mixed findings is Weiner et al. (2004) who found that aggression was *negatively* correlated with FAI for 27 women with PCOS, but positively correlated for age- and weight-matched controls. In other words, free testosterone seemed to have a calming effect on the PCOS group but not the controls. Thus, for example, State-Trait Anxiety Inventory (STAI) ratings were negatively related to the FAI for the PCOS group ($r = -0.39$, $n = 27$, $p < 0.05$) but positively correlated to the FAI in the control group ($r = 0.55$, $n = 27$, $p < 0.01$). Similar though less marked contrasts were seen for most of the State-Trait Anger Expression Inventory (STAXI) and

Aggression Questionnaire subscales. For example, for STAXI anger expression the correlation for the PCOS group was negative ($r = -0.37$, $n = 27$, $p < 0.05$) and for the controls was positive ($r = 0.37$, $n = 27$, $p < 0.05$). Archer et al. (2005) found that the correlation between testosterone and aggression was stronger in women than in men, and although the correlation is still weak, this doesn't help to explain the strange finding of Weiner et al. The conclusion of Weiner et al.—that there is a cubic (nonlinear) relationship between the FAI and mood states—seems unlikely given that this pattern of relationship was based on the combination of two different populations with significantly different FAI levels and with opposite patterns of correlations, that is, the pattern is bound to be nonlinear as the left side of the scatterplot is ascending (showing the positive relationship with FAI and disturbed mood for controls), and the right side descending (negative relationship with FAI and disturbed mood for PCOS).

So how can we best understand findings that testosterone is linked to aggression, or related constructs such as anger? A methodological issue regarding studies of PCOS (and other studies) is whether the source of aggression is testosterone, or the effects of testosterone (e.g. troubling symptoms like hirsutism), or the other effects of having PCOS (this is discussed in more detail in Chap. 7). It is easy to understand that having the troubling symptoms of PCOS might cause negative feelings, and Sills et al. (2001) found that 67% of 657 women with PCOS associated their diagnosis with 'frustration'. Elsenbruch et al. (2003) found that the significantly higher aggression scores of their PCOS group were negated when BMI was used as a covariate and Bonferroni corrections were made, which could indicate that aggression was caused by BMI (though it could also indicate that using BMI as a covariate negated the effect, i.e. a type 2 error—see Chap. 2). Note that BMI is associated with testosterone, which would make testosterone an indirect cause of aggression.

Evidence for an indirect relationship between testosterone and aggression comes from a longitudinal study of 440 transgender men (born biologically female) and transgender women. Defreyne et al. (2019) found that there was no strong evidence of a correlation between testosterone and anger scores measured on the STAXI-2 (State-Trait Anger Expression

Inventory-2). However, similar to the analysis by Barry et al. (2018), they found stronger evidence that unpleasant symptoms were associated with anger; specifically, female-to-male transsexuals who experienced menstrual spotting reported higher levels of anger.

Another weakness of the research on this topic is that although the testosterone/aggression link is strong in mice, it is much weaker in humans, and research with humans tends to yield weak associations or mixed or non-significant findings. One of the problems is that the findings are often about attitudes or traits that are only *related* to aggression, but are not aggression per se. For example, in 71 women with PCOS compared to 50 healthy control women, Asik et al. (2015) found a statistically significant positive correlation between BMI and irritable temperament. Note that irritable temperament is a cognition, and aggression a behaviour. Another aspect of this problem is that self-reports of aggression are not the same as aggressive behaviour, and research would be improved by making observations of behaviour rather than (or as well as) self-reported assessments.

Assessing aggression in humans is a vastly complex task. Although males of a given species are generally perceived as being more aggressive than females, a review by Albert et al. (1993) of the literature on aggression in humans concluded that there is little basis for the idea that testosterone causes aggression, and a meta-analysis by Book et al. (2001) found only a weak correlation ($r = 0.14$). Björkquist and Niemelä (1992) suggest that research on testosterone and aggression has tended to look for overt forms of aggression (e.g. physical rather than indirect or verbal aggression), and because men generally display the former type of aggression more than women, some researchers have concluded that men are more aggressive than women.

Testosterone causes many issues in PCOS but violence is unlikely to be one of them. The link between testosterone and aggression is strong in rodents, but weak in humans. In their review of mental health in PCOS, Himelein and Thatcher concluded that 'levels of anger and aggression do not appear to distinguish women with PCOS from control group women' (Himelein and Thatcher 2006, pp. 724–725). After more than a decade of research since then, this remains a valid conclusion if applied to testosterone, though there are some interesting findings regarding anger in PCOS (e.g. Barry et al. 2011a; Balikci et al. 2014; Gul et al. 2018) which deserve further research.

Testosterone and Depression

The evidence relating testosterone to psychological and emotional disturbance is not as clear-cut as might be expected. Some studies of the general population have observed a raised FAI in women suffering from premenstrual syndrome (PMS) (e.g. Eriksson et al. 1992), whereas other studies have found that androgen levels were not significantly different in women with PMS compared to women without PMS (e.g. Rubinow and Schmidt 1989).

Although some studies have found evidence that testosterone or other androgens are correlated with depression, the weight of evidence is that the relationship is not directly causal. Weiner et al. (2004) reported a nonlinear correlation between testosterone and depression; this study had a small sample size and the finding may have been due to chance and is unlikely to be of clinical relevance. Moran et al. (2012) found that, using a regression model controlling for BMI and other PCOS symptoms, the FAI predicted depression in PCOS. However, because the study was small (54 women with PCOS) and this correlation has not been replicated, the finding may simply be due to chance. Another study (Annagür et al. 2013) found that the adrenal androgen dehydroepiandrosterone sulphate (DHEAS) was higher in PCOS patients with clinical anxiety or depression than in controls, but this finding is less remarkable when the fact that DHEAS is produced by the adrenal glands is taken into consideration, which means that distress will increase DHEAS levels (Barry et al. 2017). Similarly, the finding by Klimczak et al. (2015) of higher adrenal androgens (DHEAS and androstenedione) in depressed women is, in the absence of a similar finding for testosterone ($p = 0.237$) or the free androgen index ($p = 0.307$), supportive of the view that testosterone has no direct impact on mood in PCOS. Indeed, the more likely explanation for the findings of Annagür et al. (2013) and Klimczak et al.

(2015) is that distress caused the increase in adrenal androgens, not vice versa. Because adrenal androgen can be converted to testosterone, a similar explanation might apply to the meta-regression finding of Cooney et al. (2017)—of higher free testosterone (but not total testosterone) in women with PCOS and anxiety, but not those with depression.

An interesting question is whether anti-androgen medication has an impact on depression in PCOS. Barnard et al. (2007) found that two-thirds of women with PCOS rated themselves on the Zung depression scale (Zung 1965) as experiencing mild depression or worse, compared to less than one-third of healthy controls. The rates were similar regardless of whether the women were taking anti-androgen medication (e.g. contraceptive pill) or not, in both the PCOS and control groups, suggesting that either the anti-androgens did not alter androgen levels or androgen levels did not affect depression levels.

Overall, the evidence suggests that depression is unlikely to be caused directly by testosterone (Barry et al. 2011a, 2018; Pastore et al. 2011; Rahiminejad et al. 2014; Batool et al. 2016; Enjezab et al. 2017; Borghi et al. 2018), and there is evidence that distress is more likely due to a negative appraisal of the symptoms of PCOS (see Chap. 7 on the psychobiological pathways in PCOS). Barry et al. (2011a) found that in women with PCOS testosterone was not generally correlated with mood states. *R square change* analysis of this data by Barry et al. (2018) found that testosterone explained only 4% of neuroticism scoring. In contrast, the quality of life impact of hirsutism explained 16% of scoring in neuroticism, quality of life for acne explained 13% of scoring in neuroticism, and quality of life for menstrual problems explained 10% of scoring in neuroticism; these three quality of life subscales statistically combined explained 25% of scoring in neuroticism. This pattern was similar when anxiety and depression were the dependent variables. Thus mood disturbance in PCOS is likely to be partly due to the fact that testosterone causes distressing physical symptoms (skin problems, subfertility, etc.), which in turn have a negative impact on mood.

Is the Testosterone-Aggression Link in Humans Just a Placebo Effect?

From the findings of research presented above, we can see there isn't much evidence for an effect of testosterone on aggression. However the idea persists in the popular mind that testosterone causes aggression, so much that it has even been used successfully in a court of law to avoid a conviction for domestic violence (Dunphy 2018, described above).

In more recent times researchers have come to understand testosterone in humans not so much as a promoter of aggression, but as a promoter of social status. In their review of studies of the effect of testosterone in social interactions, Eisenegger et al. (2011) concluded that testosterone motivates people to engage in dominance behaviour, with the aim of achieving and maintaining social status. The behaviours are usually not physically aggressive, though they might include intimidating non-verbal communication, such as staring.

One of the most interesting topics in psychology and medicine is the placebo effect. The placebo effect is when someone experiences benefits from an inert treatment that can't be attributed to properties of the treatment. The nocebo effect is a negative version of this, where someone experiences, for example, unpleasant side effects from an inert treatment which can't be attributed to the properties of the treatment. There is evidence that the popular misconception regarding testosterone and aggression in humans can create a nocebo effect, where people become more antisocial. A very interesting double-blind study of 60 healthy women found that those who were administered testosterone showed no more antisocial behaviour compared to women who were administered a placebo (Eisenegger et al. 2010). Fascinatingly, however, women who *believed* they had been administered testosterone showed more negative behaviours than those who *believed* they had received the placebo. This study demonstrates the power of false belief, and implies that people tend to have a negative conception of the effects of testosterone. It would be interesting to replicate this study in a male group to see whether the same nocebo effect occurs.

Testosterone as a Prosocial Hormone

We have seen that testosterone can have some positive effects, in terms of libido and cognition. There is also a strong case for seeing testosterone as a hormone that promotes sociability. For example, in a classic study of healthy men and women, Dabbs et al. (1997) found that those with higher levels of naturally occurring testosterone experienced more 'restless energy'. This energy spurred them to socialise with friends and engage in activities with a proactive intensity.

But testosterone is not just a feel-good hormone; it can even induce prosocial behaviour by—paradoxically—making people more competitive to be altruistic or cooperative (Roberts 1998). This is said to have evolved as a strategy used by early humans as an alternative to competing through displays of aggression. In modern times we might see examples of competitive altruism in behaviours such as giving large donations to charity, an act which will no doubt be impressive to many people, including potential romantic partners. Such altruistic behaviour can also be seen as displays that demonstrate higher status (Barry and Owens 2019). Similarly, it has been found that men who are given a testosterone supplement are less likely to lie, possibly because liars are considered untrustworthy, and thus less likely to win friends or romantic partners (Wibral et al. 2012).

There is also some interesting evidence that testosterone increases as a *result* of winning in competitive encounters, both in humans (e.g. Booth et al. 1989) and in non-human primates (e.g. Bernstein et al. 1983), and that motivation before a competition is also associated with rising testosterone (Salvador et al. 2003). This evidence reverses our usual notion of the causality of testosterone and psychology, something explored further in Chap. 7.

Of course all of the positive benefits of testosterone must be weighed against the potential negative impacts. The negative impacts are well known to women with PCOS, and include fertility problems, weight gain, and skin problems. However considering the evidence explored so far in this book (and in later chapters) it is reasonable to hypothesise that women with higher testosterone levels who either (a) don't get the distressing physiological effects of testosterone or (b) do get the physiological effects, but aren't distressed by them, might get some benefits from testosterone.

Conclusion

In conclusion, we can see that although testosterone is a problem in PCOS, it is not inevitably a problem. It's normal for women to have small amounts of testosterone, but it's only when this level is too much or too little, and becomes imbalanced in relation to estradiol, that we see problems. Even then, the problems—at least in terms of psychology—might not be as bad as we think. Indeed, as suggested in Chap. 7, the evidence tends to suggest that the direct effects of testosterone are benign or beneficial, and it is mainly the indirect effects (i.e. when testosterone causes physiological changes, which are perceived as distressing) that are problematic. In cases of aggression in humans, testosterone is only one of several variables that might contribute to that disturbance. It seems likely that some of the anger and frustration of women with PCOS comes from having to deal with a distressing condition for which there is no cure and limited support or understanding.

References

Agrawal, R., Sharma, S., Bekir, J., Conway, G., Bailey, J., Balen, A. H., & Prelevic, G. (2004). Prevalence of polycystic ovaries and polycystic ovary syndrome in lesbian women compared with heterosexual women. *Fertility and Sterility, 82*(5), 1352–1357.

Albert, D. J., Walsh, M. L., & Jonik, R. H. (1993). Aggression in humans: What is its biological foundation? *Neuroscience & Biobehavioral Reviews, 17*(4), 405–425.

Aleman, A., Bronk, E., Kessels, R. P., Koppeschaar, H. P., & van Honk, J. (2004). A single administration of testosterone improves visuospatial ability in young women. *Psychoneuroendocrinology, 29*(5), 612–617.

Annagür, B. B., Tazegül, A., Uguz, F., Kerimoglu, Ö. S., Tekinarslan, E., & Celik, Ç. (2013). Biological correlates of major depression and generalized anxiety disorder in women with polycystic ovary syndrome. *Journal of Psychosomatic Research, 74*(3), 244–247.

Archer, J., Graham-Kevan, N., & Davies, M. (2005). Testosterone and aggression: A reanalysis of Book, Starzyk, and Quinsey's (2001) study. *Aggression and Violent Behavior, 10*(2), 241–261.

Asik, M., Altinbas, K., Eroglu, M., Karaahmet, E., Erbag, G., Ertekin, H., & Sen, H. (2015). Evaluation of affective temperament and anxiety–depression levels of patients with polycystic ovary syndrome. *Journal of Affective Disorders, 185*, 214–218.

Astapova, O., Minor, B. M., & Hammes, S. R. (2019). Physiological and pathological androgen actions in the ovary. *Endocrinology, 160*(5), 1166–1174.

Azziz, R., Carmina, E., Dewailly, D., Diamanti-Kandarakis, E., Escobar-Morreale, H. F., Futterweit, W., … Witchel, S. F. (2009). The Androgen Excess and PCOS Society criteria for the polycystic ovary syndrome: The complete task force report. *Fertility and Sterility, 91*(2), 456–488.

Baba, T., Endo, T., Honnma, H., Kitajima, Y., Hayashi, T., Ikeda, H., … Saito, T. (2006). Association between polycystic ovary syndrome and female-to-male transsexuality. *Human Reproduction, 22*(4), 1011–1016.

Balen, A. H., Schachter, M. E., Montgomery, D., Reid, R. W., & Jacobs, H. S. (1993). Polycystic ovaries are a common finding in untreated female to male transsexuals. *Clinical Endocrinology, 38*(3), 325–329.

Balikci, A., Erdem, M., KESKIN, U., Zincir, S. B., Guelsuen, M., Oezcelik, F., … Erguen, A. (2014). Depression, anxiety, and anger in patients with polycystic ovary syndrome. *Nöro Psikiyatri Arşivi, 51*(4), 328.

Barnard, L., Ferriday, D., Guenther, N., Strauss, B., Balen, A. H., & Dye, L. (2007). Quality of life and psychological well being in polycystic ovary syndrome. *Human Reproduction, 22*(8), 2279–2286.

Barry, J. A., & Owens, R. (2019). From fetuses to boys to men: The impact of testosterone on male lifespan development. In *The Palgrave handbook of male psychology and mental health* (pp. 3–24). Cham: Palgrave Macmillan.

Barry, J. A., Hardiman, P. J., Saxby, B. K., & Kuczmierczyk, A. (2011a). Testosterone and mood dysfunction in women with polycystic ovarian syndrome compared to subfertile controls. *Journal of Psychosomatic Obstetrics and Gynecology, 32*(2), 104–111.

Barry, J. A., Hardiman, P. J., Siddiqui, M. R., & Thomas, M. (2011b). Meta-analysis of sex difference in testosterone levels in umbilical cord blood. *Journal of Obstetrics and Gynaecology, 31*(8), 697–702.

Barry, J. A., Parekh, H. S. K., & Hardiman, P. J. (2013). Visual-spatial cognition in women with polycystic ovarian syndrome: The role of androgens. *Human Reproduction, 28*(10), 2832–2837.

Barry, J. A., Leite, N., Sivarajah, N., Keevil, B., Owen, L., Miranda, L. C., … Hardiman, P. (2017). Relaxation and guided imagery significantly reduces androgen levels and distress in polycystic ovary syndrome: Pilot study. *Contemporary Hypnosis and Integrative Therapy, 32*(1), 21–29.

Barry, J. A., Qu, F., & Hardiman, P. J. (2018). An exploration of the hypothesis that testosterone is implicated in the psychological functioning of women with polycystic ovary syndrome (PCOS). *Medical Hypotheses, 110*, 42–45.

Batool, S., ul ain Ahmed, F., Ambreen, A., Sheikh, A., & Faryad, N. (2016). Depression and anxiety in women with polycystic ovary syndrome and its biochemical associates. *Journal of South Asian Federation of Obstetrics and Gynaecology, 8*(1), 44–47.

Bernstein, I. S., Gordon, T. P., & Rose, R. M. (1983). The interaction of hormones, behavior, and social context in nonhuman primates. In *Hormones and aggressive behavior* (pp. 535–561). Boston: Springer.

Björkqvist, K., & Niemelä, P. (1992). New trends in the study of female aggression. In K. Björkqvist & P. Niemelä (Eds.), *Of mice and women: Aspects of female aggression* (pp. 3–16). San Diego, CA, US: Academic Press.

Boehmer, U., Bowen, D. J., & Bauer, G. R. (2007). Overweight and obesity in sexual-minority women: Evidence from population-based data. *American Journal of Public Health, 97*(6), 1134–1140.

Book, A. S., Starzyk, K. B., & Quinsey, V. L. (2001). The relationship between testosterone and aggression: A meta-analysis. *Aggression and Violent Behavior, 6*(6), 579–599.

Booth, A., Shelley, G., Mazur, A., Tharp, G., & Kittok, R. (1989). Testosterone, and winning and losing in human competition. *Hormones and Behavior, 23*, 556–571.

Booth, A., Granger, D. A., Mazur, A., & Kivlighan, K. T. (2006). Testosterone and social behavior. *Social Forces, 85*(1), 167–191.

Borghi, L., Leone, D., Vegni, E., Galiano, V., Lepadatu, C., Sulpizio, P., & Garzia, E. (2018). Psychological distress, anger and quality of life in polycystic ovary syndrome: Associations with biochemical, phenotypical and socio-demographic factors. *Journal of Psychosomatic Obstetrics and Gynecology, 39*(2), 128–137.

Bosinski, H. A., Peter, M., Bonatz, G., Arndt, R., Heidenreich, M., Sippell, W. G., & Wille, R. (1997). A higher rate of hyperandrogenic disorders in female-to-male transsexuals. *Psychoneuroendocrinology, 22*(5), 361–380.

Cesta, C. E., Månsson, M., Palm, C., Lichtenstein, P., Iliadou, A. N., & Landén, M. (2016). Polycystic ovary syndrome and psychiatric disorders: Co-morbidity and heritability in a nationwide Swedish cohort. *Psychoneuroendocrinology, 73*, 196–203.

Chen, C. H., Wang, P. H., Hsieh, M. T., Tzeng, C. R., Wu, Y. H., Lee, C. S., ... Chang, H. Y. (2014). Sexual orientations of women with polycystic ovary syndrome: Clinical observation in Taiwan. *Taiwanese Journal of Obstetrics and Gynecology, 53*(4), 542–546.

Cooney, L. G., Lee, I., Sammel, M. D., & Dokras, A. (2017). High prevalence of moderate and severe depressive and anxiety symptoms in polycystic ovary syndrome: A systematic review and meta-analysis. *Human Reproduction, 32*(5), 1075–1091.

Dabbs, J. M., Jr., Strong, R., & Milun, R. (1997). Exploring the mind of testosterone: A beeper study. *Journal of Research in Personality, 31*(4), 577–587.

Davis, S. (2001). Testosterone treatment: Psychological and physical effects in postmenopausal women. *American Society for Reproductive Medicine: Menopausal Medicine, 9*(2).

De Sutter, P., Dutré, T., Vanden Meerschaut, F., Stuyver, I., Van Maele, G., & Dhont, M. (2008). PCOS in lesbian and heterosexual women treated with artificial donor insemination. *Reproductive Biomedicine Online, 17*(3), 398–402.

Defreyne, J., Kreukels, B., T'Sjoen, G., Stahporsius, A., Den Heijer, M., Heylens, G., & Elaut, E. (2019). No correlation between serum testosterone levels and state-level anger intensity in transgender people: Results from the European Network for the Investigation of Gender Incongruence. *Hormones and Behavior, 110*, 29–39.

Dittman, R. W., Kappes, M. E., & Kappes, M. H. (1992). Sexual behaviour and adolescent and adult females with congenital adrenal hyperplasia. *Psychoneuroendocrinology, 17*, 153–170.

Dunphy, L. (2018, January 18). *Lesbian mum who viciously beat bride walks free after telling court she has high levels of "male hormones"*. Retrieved from https://www.mirror.co.uk/news/uk-news/lesbian-mum-who-viciously-beat-11872183#ICID=sharebar_twitter.

Eisenegger, C., Naef, M., Snozzi, R., Heinrichs, M., & Fehr, E. (2010). Prejudice and truth about the effect of testosterone on human bargaining behaviour. *Nature, 463*(7279), 356.

Eisenegger, C., Haushofer, J., & Fehr, E. (2011). The role of testosterone in social interaction. *Trends in Cognitive Sciences, 15*(6), 263–271.

Elsenbruch, S., Hahn, S., Kowalsky, D., Offner, A. H., Schedlowski, M., Mann, K., & Janssen, O. E. (2003). Quality of life, psychosocial well-being, and sexual satisfaction in women with polycystic ovary syndrome. *The Journal of Clinical Endocrinology and Metabolism, 88*, 5801–5807.

Enjezab, B., Eftekhar, M., & Ghadiri-Anari, A. (2017). Association between severity of depression and clinico-biochemical markers of polycystic ovary syndrome. *Electronic Physician, 9*(11), 5820.

Ercan, C. M., Coksuer, H., Aydogan, U., Alanbay, I., Keskin, U., Karasahin, K. E., & Baser, I. (2013). Sexual dysfunction assessment and hormonal correlations in patients with polycystic ovary syndrome. *International Journal of Impotence Research, 25*, 127–132.

Eriksson, E., Sundblad, C., Lisjö, P., Modigh, K., & Andersch, B. (1992). Serum levels of androgens are higher in women with premenstrual irritability and dysphoria than in controls. *Psychoneuroendocrinology, 17*(2–3), 195–204.

Futterweit, W., Weiss, R. A., & Fagerstrom, R. M. (1986). Endocrine evaluation of forty female-to-male transsexuals: Increased frequency of polycystic ovarian disease in female transsexualism. *Archives of Sexual Behavior, 15*(1), 69–78.

Gallinelli, A., Matteo, M. L., Volpe, A., & Facchinetti, F. (2000). Autonomic and neuroendocrine responses to stress in patients with functional hypothalamic secondary amenorrhea. *Fertility and Sterility, 73*(4), 812–816.

Gul, A., Gul, H., Ergur, A. T., & Ozen, N. E. (2018). Anxiety-anger relationship in hyperandrogenemia: A comparative study with polycystic ovary syndrome (PCOS) and healthy control adolescents. *Journal of Mood Disorders, 8*(1), 26–31.

Hahn, S., Janssen, O. E., Tan, S., Pleger, K., Mann, K., Schedlowski, M., … Elsenbruch, S. (2005). Clinical and psychological correlates of quality-of-life in polycystic ovary syndrome. *European Journal of Endocrinology, 153*, 853–860.

Himelein, M. J., & Thatcher, S. S. (2006). Depression and body image among women with polycystic ovary syndrome. *Journal of Health Psychology, 11*(4), 613–625.

Klimczak, D., Szlendak-Sauer, K., & Radowicki, S. (2015). Depression in relation to biochemical parameters and age in women with polycystic ovary syndrome. *European Journal of Obstetrics & Gynecology and Reproductive Biology, 184*, 43–47.

Legro, R. S., Schlaff, W. D., Diamond, M. P., Coutifaris, C., Casson, P. R., Brzyski, R. G., … Ohl, D. (2010). Total testosterone assays in women with polycystic ovary syndrome: Precision and correlation with hirsutism. *The Journal of Clinical Endocrinology & Metabolism, 95*(12), 5305–5313.

Lujan, M. E., & Mergler, R. J. (2015). Cognitive function in women with polycystic ovary syndrome (PCOS): Impact of reproductive and metabolic factors. *Fertility and Sterility, 104*(3), e129.

Manlove, A. H., Guillermo, C., & Gray, P. B. (2008). Do women with polycystic ovary syndrome (PCOS) report differences in sex-typed behavior as children and adolescents?: Results of a pilot study. *Annals of Human Biology, 35*(6), 584–595.

McCook, J. G. (2002). *The influence of hyperandrogenism, obesity and infertility on the psychosocial health and wellbeing of women with polycystic ovary syndrome.* Unpublished doctoral dissertation, University of Michigan.

Monzani, F., Pucci, F., Caraccio, N., Bagnolesi, A., Molli, D., Fenu, A., & Prunetti, C. (1994). Psychological and psychopathological correlates in the polycystic ovary syndrome (PCOS). *Medicina Psicosomatica, 39*, 225–236.

Moran, L. J., Deeks, A. A., Gibson-Helm, M. E., & Teede, H. J. (2012). Psychological parameters in the reproductive phenotypes of polycystic ovary syndrome. *Human Reproduction, 27*, 2082–2088.

Nathorst-Böös, J., Flöter, A., Jarkander-Rolff, M., Carlström, K., & Von Schoultz, B. (2006). Treatment with percutaneous testosterone gel in postmenopausal women with decreased libido–effects on sexuality and psychological general well-being. *Maturitas, 53*(1), 11–18.

Nordqvist, S., Sydsjö, G., Lampic, C., Åkerud, H., Elenis, E., & Skoog Svanberg, A. (2014). Sexual orientation of women does not affect outcome of fertility treatment with donated sperm. *Human Reproduction, 29*(4), 704–711.

Pastore, L. M., Patrie, J. T., Morris, W. L., Dalal, P., & Bray, M. J. (2011). Depression symptoms and body dissatisfaction association among polycystic ovary syndrome women. *Journal of Psychosomatic Research, 71*(4), 270–276.

Peters, M., Laeng, B., Latham, K., Jackson, M., Zaiyouna, R., & Richardson, C. (1995). A redrawn Vandenberg and Kuse mental rotations test-different versions and factors that affect performance. *Brain and Cognition, 28*(1), 39–58.

Pintzka, C. W., Evensmoen, H. R., Lehn, H., & Håberg, A. K. (2016). Changes in spatial cognition and brain activity after a single dose of testosterone in healthy women. *Behavioural Brain Research, 298*, 78–90.

Rahiminejad, M. E., Moaddab, A., Rabiee, S., Esna-Ashari, F., Borzouei, S., & Hosseini, S. M. (2014). The relationship between clinicobiochemical markers and depression in women with polycystic ovary syndrome. *Iranian Journal of Reproductive Medicine, 12*(12), 811.

Rasgon, N. L., Rao, R. C., Hwang, S., Altshuler, L. L., Elman, S., Zuckerbrow-Miller, J., & Korenman, S. G. (2003). Depression in women with polycystic ovary syndrome: Clinical and biochemical correlates. *Journal of Affective Disorders, 74*(3), 299–304.

Rellini, A. H., Stratton, N., Tonani, S., Santamaria, V., Brambilla, E., & Nappi, R. E. (2013). Differences in sexual desire between women with clinical versus biochemical signs of hyperandrogenism in polycystic ovarian syndrome. *Hormones and Behavior, 63*, 65–71.

Roberts, G. (1998). Competitive altruism: From reciprocity to the handicap principle. *Proceedings of the Royal Society of London B: Biological Sciences, 265*(1394), 427–431.

Robinson, K., Galloway, K. Y., Bewley, S., & Meads, C. (2017). Lesbian and bisexual women's gynaecological conditions: A systematic review and exploratory meta-analysis. *BJOG: An International Journal of Obstetrics & Gynaecology, 124*(3), 381–392.

Roche Diagnostics. (2000). Elecsys Testosterone Product Information. Retrieved May 5, 2010, from http://www.roche-diagnostics.ch/resource.php?id=Resourcefile-37084379e9754cf58.

Rosner, W., Auchus, R. J., Azziz, R., Sluss, P. M., & Raff, H. (2007). Position statement: Utility, limitations, and pitfalls in measuring testosterone: An endocrine society position statement. *Journal of Clinical Endocrinology & Metabolism, 92*, 405–413.

Rubinow, D. R., & Schmidt, P. J. (1989). Models for the development and expression of symptoms in premenstrual syndrome. *Psychiatric Clinics, 12*(1), 53–68.

Salvador, A., Suay, F., Gonzalez-Bono, E., & Serrano, M. A. (2003). Anticipatory cortisol, testosterone and psychological responses to judo competition in young men. *Psychoneuroendocrinology, 28*(3), 364–375.

Schattmann, L., & Sherwin, B. B. (2007). Testosterone levels and cognitive functioning in women with polycystic ovary syndrome and in healthy young women. *Hormones and Behavior, 51*(5), 587–596.

Schüring, A. N., Nolte, S., Fobker, M., Kannenberg, F., & Nofer, J. R. (2016). Head-to-head assessment of diagnostic performance of testosterone immunoassays in patients with polycystic ovary syndrome. *Journal of Clinical Laboratory Analysis, 30*(5), 479–484.

Shepard, R. N., & Metzler, J. (1971). Mental rotation of three-dimensional objects. *Science, 171*(3972), 701–703.

Sills, E. S., Perloe, M., Tucker, M. J., Kaplan, C. R., Genton, M. G., & Schattman, G. L. (2001). Diagnostic and treatment characteristics of polycystic ovary syndrome: Descriptive measurements of patient perception and awareness from 657 confidential self-reports. *BMC Women's Health, 1*(1), 3.

Smith, A. M., Rissel, C. E., Richters, J., Grulich, A. E., & de Visser, R. O. (2003). Sex in Australia: Sexual identity, sexual attraction and sexual experience among a representative sample of adults. *Australian and New Zealand Journal of Public Health, 27*(2), 138–145.

Smith, H. A., Markovic, N., Matthews, A. K., Danielson, M. E., Kalro, B. N., Youk, A. O., & Talbott, E. O. (2011). A comparison of polycystic ovary syndrome and related factors between lesbian and heterosexual women. *Women's Health Issues, 21*(3), 191–198.

Taher, S., Rothon, C., & Panay, N. (2008). Testosterone gel and improvement in libido, psychological state and general wellbeing in natural and surgical post-menopausal women: P3. 24. *Bjog: An International Journal of Obstetrics and Gynaecology, 115*(187).

Udiawar, M. (2017). *Cardiometabolic and neuroimaging correlates of cognitive function in polycystic ovary syndrome.* Doctoral dissertation, Cardiff University.

Weiner, C. L., Primeau, M., & Ehrmann, D. A. (2004). Androgens and mood dysfunction in women: Comparison of women with polycystic ovarian syndrome to healthy controls. *Psychosomatic Medicine, 66*(3), 356–362.

Wibral, M., Dohmen, T., Klingmüller, D., Weber, B., & Falk, A. (2012). Testosterone administration reduces lying in men. *PLoS One, 7*(10), e46774.

Zucker, K. J., Bradley, S. J., Oliver, G., Blake, J., Fleming, S., & Hood, J. (1996). Psychosexual development of women with congenital adrenal hyperplasia. *Hormones and Behavior, 30*(4), 300–318.

Zung, W. W. (1965). A self-rating depression scale. *Archives of General Psychiatry, 12*(1), 63–70.

5

Insulin Resistance, Diabetes, Mood and Binge Eating

Abstract Although testosterone is often seen as the main hormone of interest in PCOS, insulin is also a key player. Indeed in some ways insulin is more significant to PCOS than is testosterone, though perhaps less dramatic in its impact, especially when it comes to psychology. However, the most obvious effect that insulin has on psychology is through hypoglycaemia—low blood sugar—and this phenomenon possibly makes a substantial contribution to anxiety, depression, and neuroticism in PCOS. This chapter explores the role of insulin in PCOS and studies how it is related to testosterone, obesity, and binge eating.

Keywords Insulin • Diabetes • Hypoglycaemia • Depression • Metformin

Introduction

According to Diamanti-Kandarakis and Christakou, international experts on PCOS: 'Insulin resistance refers to the state, wherein insulin action is insufficient to accomplish the metabolic demands of peripheral tissues,

© The Author(s) 2019
J. A. Barry, *Psychological Aspects of Polycystic Ovary Syndrome*,
https://doi.org/10.1007/978-3-030-30290-0_5

despite the increased amounts of insulin secreted in the circulation. However, this is only an approximate description of this disorder. Insulin resistance encompasses an elaborate clinical, pathophysiologic, and molecular spectrum, and therefore, a well-established definition remains elusive' (Diamanti-Kandarakis and Christakou 2009, p. 35). Other PCOS experts such as Ovalle and Azziz say that 'Insulin resistance is considered to be a fundamental defect in patients with type 2 diabetes mellitus … Type 2 diabetes mellitus is a heterogeneous metabolic disorder characterized by hyperglycaemia resulting from a combination of resistance to insulin action and an inadequate compensatory insulin secretory response' (Ovalle and Azziz 2002, pp. 1095–1099). These definitions will sound complex to the non-endocrinologist, but in very simple terms, this means that insulin resistance occurs when the cells of the human body stop reacting to the presence of insulin, even if the body produces more insulin in an effort to get a reaction. If this situation continues over a number of years, this results in a condition called type 2 diabetes mellitus (usually referred to as type 2 diabetes).

Why are these phenomena important in a book on the psychological aspects of PCOS? Well firstly, insulin resistance and type 2 diabetes are more common in women with PCOS than in healthy women. Secondly, type 2 diabetes is associated with fatigue and low mood (as described later), because insulin has a key role in helping the body use glucose to give us energy.

The link between PCOS and type 2 diabetes has been known since 1980 (Burghen et al. 1980). Type 2 diabetes is a serious public health issue, which requires a massive annual budget (Ding et al. 2018). Insulin resistance is a key pathophysiological feature of PCOS, contributing not only to type 2 diabetes, but to raised testosterone, reproductive issues, and even cardiometabolic risk (Moran et al. 2010). Prospective clinical studies in the US have found the prevalence of type 2 diabetes in women with PCOS is 7.5%–10%, which is about 10 times higher than what is seen in healthy women of a similar age (Farrell and Antoni 2010). An assessment of a large UK primary care database found that the prevalence of type 2 diabetes is 26.5% for women diagnosed with PCOS, or present in those with symptoms that suggest undiagnosed PCOS (Ding et al. 2018). The apparent difference in rates between the US and UK (10% vs 26.5%) is probably due to methodological differences: the UK study included a general population sample rather than women recruited from a clinic, and included women whose symptoms suggested having PCOS rather than an actual diagnosis. Also the UK study made the estimate using Bayesian methods, and did not control for ethnicity, though diabetes varies by ethnic group (Zhao and Qiao 2013).

In Iran, a study of 178 women with PCOS (mean ± SD age 26.4 ± 8.5) and 1524 healthy control-group women (aged 28.9 ± 8.6) found an incidence rate of diabetes of 13.4 in PCOS women and 4.2 in controls (Jaliseh et al. 2017). Participants were followed over a median of around 13 years, and—in some good news for women with PCOS—it was found that the risk of diabetes in PCOS decreased with age in PCOS, probably because women with PCOS have learned to successfully use medication and lifestyle modifications.

The Role of Obesity in Diabetes

Insulin resistance is sometimes seen as a precursor to type 2 diabetes. It can be genetic, or the result of lifestyle characterised by a lack of exercise, high-carbohydrate diet, and stress. The term 'diathesis-stress' is used to convey the idea that type 2 diabetes can be the result of both nature and nurture; those with a genetic vulnerability to developing type 2 diabetes will only do so if they experience the 'stressor' of an unhealthy lifestyle.

Insulin resistance is caused when the number of insulin receptors on cell wall is reduced, and in PCOS, this reduction can be up to 75% (reduced from roughly 20,000 receptors to 5000 receptors). This means that the ability of serum glucose (blood sugar) to enter the cell to be converted to energy is reduced, and must instead remain in the bloodstream until converted by the liver into fat. The accumulation of fat leads to obesity, which in itself can contribute to PCOS (Sam 2007). A meta-analysis by Moran et al. (2010) found that women with PCOS had an elevated prevalence of type 2 diabetes, impaired glucose tolerance, and metabolic syndrome. The greater prevalence of diabetes (OR = 4.43) was seen even after BMI was controlled for by matching (OR = 4.0), suggesting that obesity alone does not explain the higher prevalence of diabetes in PCOS.

Carrying weight on the stomach rather than on the hips is known as central (or android) obesity, and is related to elevated androgen levels. Although insulin resistance occurs in non-obese women (Dunaif and Book 1997), non-diabetic women with central obesity typically have elevated androgens, IR, and hyperinsulinaemia (elevated blood insulin levels) (Kissebah et al. 1989).

Is Insulin More Significant in PCOS Than Testosterone?

Insulin plays an important role in PCOS, though whether it is more important than testosterone is open to debate (Azziz et al. 2008) and may depend on the PCOS phenotype in question (see Chap. 1) or the level at which etiology is being considered. There is a positive correlation between testosterone and insulin levels in women with PCOS (Buffington et al. 1991). Given that testosterone is considered a central feature of PCOS, it is interesting that elevated testosterone is often seen as caused by elevated insulin (Farrell and Antoni 2010). This direction of causality is unexpected for many non-endocrinologists, but makes more sense when you consider that insulin-sensitising drugs such as metformin can reduce hyperandrogenism (Moghetti et al. 2000), but anti-androgen drugs don't generally improve insulin resistance (Diamanti-Kandarakis et al. 1995). However nothing is simple in the endocrine system and the reality is that insulin and testosterone are in a cyclical relationship: insulin promotes testosterone, testosterone promotes visceral fat and insulin resistance, and this elevates insulin levels (Stanley and Misra 2008). (See also Fig. 7.1, Chap. 7.)

There are at least two ways in which insulin contributes to testosterone levels. One is by reducing SHBG levels (see Chap. 4), which means that testosterone is more able to exert its androgenic effects (Nestler 1991). The other pathway is via the ovaries: insulin causes androgen production in the ovaries (Yen 1991). Despite insulin resistance often being a feature of PCOS, the ovaries in PCOS remain sensitive to insulin; there is as yet no explanation for this phenomenon (Diamanti-Kandarakis et al. 2008).

Depression and Insulin Resistance in PCOS

There is some interesting evidence that insulin resistance is associated with depression in PCOS. Most studies of PCOS measure insulin resistance using the Homeostasis Model Assessment Insulin Resistance index (HOMA-IR), which is calculated from the results of a fasting insulin test and a fasting glucose test. Cinar et al. (2011) found that depression scores are correlated with insulin resistance, lipid parameters, and the severity of metabolic syndrome in PCOS. In 71 women with PCOS compared to 50 healthy control-group women, Asik et al. (2015) found a statistically significant positive correlation between insulin and HADS depression scores in patients with PCOS. Batool et al. (2016) found that although there was no significant difference in testosterone or adrenal androgens between depressed and non-depressed women with PCOS, there was higher fasting insulin levels and impaired fasting glucose among the depressed group. In a study of 301 women with PCOS, Greenwood et al. (2015) found that depression was partly explained by insulin resistance, independent of BMI. They replicated this finding in a larger sample of 738 women with PCOS, concluding that 'Insulin resistance has a strong and independent association with depression in PCOS' (Greenwood et al. 2018, p. 27).

Not all studies have found this association, though of course 'absence of evidence is not evidence of absence'. Ozdemir et al. (2016) assessed BDI scores in 69 patients with PCOS and 49 healthy controls. They found no link between insulin resistance and atypical depression (characterised by symptoms such as weight gain and fatigue). Enjezab et al. (2015) did not find a significant relationship between depression scores and physiological variables (BMI, insulin resistance, or testosterone) in 62 women with PCOS. This lack of significance was not due to the sample size, because although the correlation for BMI was in the expected direction ($r = 0.2$, $p < 0.10$), the relationship with insulin resistance was in the opposite direction to that expected ($r = -0.2$, $p < 0.09$). However these are bivariate correlations, and thus do not take into account other factors that might influence the correlation, such as metformin use and exercise, which did not appear to be controlled in this study.

Erensoy et al. (2019) gave 1500 mg of metformin to 44 women with PCOS for 90 days and found significantly decreased insulin resistance and BMI. The treatment also improved depression (from BDI ~21 to ~18) and anxiety levels (from BAI ~20 to ~16). Although the changes in mood were not statistically significant, they represent changes from borderline moderate levels of mood problem to mild levels, and a larger sample size might have seen these non-trivial changes become statistically significant. What is the mechanism that connects taking metformin to improved mood? Erensoy et al. suggest that it could simply be due to improvements in weight and body image. Greenwood et al. (2015) suggest it could be that insulin resistance underlies the troubling symptoms of PCOS, or alternatively, that complex insulin-related neural phenomena may be involved. Other possibilities, related to their first suggestion, could be that insulin resistance is associated with type 2 diabetes, which is relatively common in PCOS, and is a condition that is associated with troubling symptoms (e.g. weight gain) and can be troublesome to manage (e.g. restrictive lifestyle, insulin injections). These difficulties would make the association between insulin resistance and depression understandable at face value. A pilot study of the impact of metformin on mood supports this hypothesis: Erensoy et al. (2019) assessed the impact of metformin on insulin resistance and anxiety and depression in 19 adolescents and 25 adult women with PCOS in Iran. Overall the 44 participants had significantly improved BMI, WHR, fasting blood glucose, and serum insulin. Anxiety and depression scores significantly improved too, though there were no significant improvements in testosterone, DHEAS, or lipid profile. Erensoy et al. interpreted the improvements in mood as being caused either by the improvement in BMI or by improvements in insulin sensitivity. Although the former interpretation makes sense, the experimental design (no control group, no control for effect of BMI in mood changes from baseline to post-treatment) means that we don't really know the impact of BMI. As to the latter interpretation, we have to ask what the mechanism might be; in other words, how would an improvement in insulin sensitivity lead to an improvement in anxiety and depression, independent of improvements of PCOS symptoms?

A possibility not usually considered is the impact of insulin resistance on lowering blood sugar levels, causing 'hypoglycaemia'. This explanation offers a relatively direct mechanism for the impact of insulin resistance on mood, and is explored next (and in Chap. 7).

Low Blood Sugar (Hypoglycaemia) and Mood

Although it is popularly thought that eating a sugary snack gives an energy boost, a meta-analysis of 31 studies on the impact of carbohydrate consumption on mood found that the 'sugar rush' is a myth (Mantantzis et al. 2019). In fact they found evidence instead for a 'sugar crash', characterised by greater fatigue 30 minutes after consumption, and less alertness after 60 minutes.

This is of relevance to PCOS, because Marsh et al. (2010) note that besides the more typical symptoms of PCOS, some women with PCOS claim that they experience symptoms typical of low blood glucose levels, also known as *hypoglycaemia*. These symptoms are said to be associated with certain foods and eating patterns, and even linked with a craving for sweet food or drinks. The claims of these patients are sometimes met with scepticism (in the UK at least, though some countries, such as France, are less sceptical), but an inspection of the research evidence tells us that we should be more open-minded, especially as controlling blood sugar levels is a concern for many women with PCOS—41.6% of 60 women with PCOS in a study by Kerchner et al. (2009).

Reactive (or 'postprandial') hypoglycaemia happens when blood glucose levels drop after a meal. This occurs around two to five hours after the meal, especially a meal high in carbohydrates. Signs typical of lower blood sugar in the brain (neuroglycopenia) are clumsiness, confusion, sudden weakness, and difficulty in speaking. More general autonomic symptoms are palpitations, sweating, and shivering. The general mood state of hypoglycaemia has been described as 'tense-tiredness': anxiety, low mood, and fatigue (Thayer 1987). In healthy women, there is a rate of about 12.4% of reactive hypoglycaemia (Sørensen and Johansen 2010), but in women with PCOS, the rate is much higher. In 'lean' women, the rate is 50% (Altuntas et al. 2005), and in obese women with PCOS the rate is 66% (Kasim-Karakas et al. 2007). Brand-Miller et al. (2004) describe hypoglycaemia as one of the 'subtle symptoms' of PCOS, and this may well be true. For example, fatigue is one of the most commonly reported symptoms of depression in women with PCOS (Hollinrake et al. 2007), which is the third of the 'tense-tired' signs.

Despite the known links between PCOS and depression and anxiety (two of the three 'tense-tired' symptoms) and high rates of reactive hypoglycaemia, the link between PCOS and hypoglycaemia has received surprisingly little research attention. The first study of this kind was done by Barry et al. (2011c) who conducted an online survey, assessing symptoms typical of hypoglycaemia in 24 women with PCOS, 299 healthy control-group women, and 47 women who probably had undiagnosed PCOS. After controlling for age, BMI, and eating behaviour (using matching and ANCOVA), it was found that women with PCOS reported higher scores on signs of hypoglycaemia. Although these findings are interesting, we know from Chap. 2 that BMI can't really be controlled for in studies of PCOS. Another weakness of this study is that it only assessed psychological signs of PCOS without assessing actual blood glucose levels as well. Further research on this topic is needed. This topic, potentially of importance to women with PCOS. (See also Chap. 7 on the hypothesised cause of hypoglycaemia in PCOS, and Chap. 8 regarding the low-GI diet for PCOS.)

Binge Eating in PCOS

Cesta et al. (2016) found that the chances of having any kind of eating disorder was 18% higher in women with PCOS (AOR = 1.18). Eating disorders, especially binge eating, are a serious issue in PCOS. That is because even in healthy women, just a single day of binging on high-fat foods is enough to impair glycaemic control and reduce insulin sensitivity (Taylor et al. 1999; Parry et al. 2017). The impact might potentially be even more dramatic in PCOS, where insulin resistance is already a problem. By the same token, there is some interesting evidence that overcoming bulimia can actually normalise previously polycystic ovaries in PCOS (Morgan et al. 2002).

The usual advice for PCOS patients is diet and exercise. For women who are prone to eating disorders such as anorexia, or excessive exercise, this advice can be counterproductive for obvious reasons. However, probably the most common disordered eating behaviour in PCOS is binge eating.

Binge eating behaviour is characterised by overeating, followed by feeling distressed (NHS 2017). A meta-analysis (Lee et al. 2018) of eight studies (470 women with PCOS and 390 healthy controls) found that women with PCOS had over three times the odds of being diagnosed with an eating disorder (OR 3.87). There was not enough statistical power to find statistically significant differences in subtypes of eating disorders, but in general, studies find that there is at least twice the prevalence of binge eating in PCOS women compared to other women. For example, Bernadett et al. (2016) found a 43% prevalence of binge-eating behaviour in PCOS women compared to 12.4% in other women.

In general, validated measures should be used in research. Some studies of eating behaviour in PCOS didn't use standardised eating disorder measures (e.g. Barry et al. 2011c), but even when standardised measures as used (e.g. self-report measures such as the Eating Attitudes Test-26, created by Garner et al. 1982), these are likely to be prone to 'false-positive' diagnoses (Bernadett et al. 2016). The best assessments are interview-based techniques such as the SCID (First et al. 1996) or the Eating Disorder Examination (EDE, Fairburn et al. 2008), though these are more time-consuming than self-administered questionnaires, so are less commonly used.

The cause of binge eating in PCOS is likely to be a combination of factors, the main ones being psychological factors and hormonal factors (insulin resistance and androgens).

Psychological Factors Causing Binge Eating in PCOS

The symptoms typical of PCOS can be distressing. They can impact body satisfaction and contribute to the development of binge eating (Stice and Shaw 2002), because binge eating can be a way of coping with the distress (Karacan et al. 2014; Himelein and Thatcher 2006). Paganini et al. (2018) found that increased hunger can be caused by menstrual irregularity and psychological distress, which can potentially trigger binge-eating behaviour. It is well established that women with PCOS are more prone to negative mood states than are other women (e.g. Barry et al. 2011b). Even after controlling for age and BMI, anxiety and depression are associated with greater risk of eating pathology in PCOS (Lee et al. 2017). Indeed anxiety and depression are independently predictors of eating disorders (Månson et al. 2008; Karacan et al. 2014). Negative emotions in general contribute to binge-eating behaviour (Månsson et al. 2008), and bulimia nervosa was found to be higher in PCOS even after controlling for other psychiatric disorders (Cesta et al. 2016).

Insulin Resistance and Androgens Causing Binge Eating in PCOS

Insulin resistance undoubtedly plays a role in eating disorders in PCOS, especially binge eating (Paganini et al. 2018). This is because many women with PCOS are inclined to have hypoglycaemia (i.e. low blood glucose), and when this occurs, it is not unusual to experience 'carbohydrate cravings' in order to restore glucose levels to normal (Maharaj and Amod 2009; Bartholome et al. 2006; Larsson et al. 2016). Hypoglycaemia is caused by insulin resistance because when the body's cells resist the uptake of insulin, insulin accumulates in the bloodstream, driving down levels of blood glucose (Jeanes et al. 2017; Paganini et al. 2018). This can lead to weight gain independent of lifestyle habits (Bellver et al. 2018; Diamanti-Kandarakis and Papavassiliou 2006), and can become a vicious cycle, where obesity can increase insulin resistance (Norman et al. 2004). This makes usual weight loss strategies very difficult for women with PCOS, because they don't tend to lead to enduring weight loss, unless the weight loss is such that it cures the insulin resistance. (Weight loss strategies are discussed in Chap. 8.)

In non-PCOS women with bulimia (Sundblad et al. 1994) and animal studies (Iwasa et al. 2018), androgens can be an appetite stimulant; thus, in theory, androgen might increase appetite in women with PCOS. More research is needed to establish this link in PCOS, but one small study of bulimia found that the administration of flutamide (an androgen receptor antagonist) reduced symptoms of bulimia (Sundblad et al. 2005). Furthermore, Hirschberg et al. (2004) found that women with PCOS have reduced secretion of cholecystokinin, a peptide that signals satiety, which is likely to impact appetite regulation.

Medication for Insulin Resistance

Drug treatment of PCOS usually aims to reduce testosterone levels—either indirectly by using the insulin sensitiser metformin, or directly by using anti-androgens or contraceptives that have an anti-androgenic effect (e.g. Dianette or spironolactone). Metformin is also used with the primary aim of reducing insulin resistance in PCOS, as insulin resistance is not uncommonly comorbid with PCOS (Dunaif et al. 1989). Hunter and Sterrett (2000) suggest that metformin reduces testosterone levels and restores normal menstrual cyclicity. Pasquali et al. (2000) found that metformin decreased testosterone levels in women with PCOS, and that both women with PCOS and healthy controls treated with metformin experienced a reduction in their BMI. In a case study of a woman with untreated PCOS and major depression, Rasgon et al. (2002) found that treatment with metformin and spironolactone (an anti-androgen also used for liver and heart complaints) resolved both the depression and PCOS. Metformin may also lead to weight reduction, decrease in lipid levels, decrease in blood pressure, and restoration of a normal menstrual functioning. Although metformin can cause gastrointestinal side effects in the first few weeks of use (Fruzzetti et al. 2017), Muth et al. (2004) report that they found it difficult to recruit women with PCOS on metformin to a study that required them to stop taking metformin: 77% of the 22 women he approached at the Glasgow Royal Infirmary refused. So, in this small sample at least, there was support for metformin from PCOS patients, suggesting that the side effects do not discourage adherence.

A potential alternative to metformin is inositol, which is part of the vitamin B complex, and has more recently begun to be used as insulin sensitiser in the treatment of PCOS. Human adults consume approximately one gram of inositol, mainly MYO, per day in different biochemical forms. Circulating free MYO is taken up by most tissues, and inositol uptake is inhibited by glucose. A systematic review of RCTs of myo-inositol in women with PCOS (Unfer et al. 2012) found strong evidence of MYO effectiveness, and recommends four grams daily as the maximum dose with minimal side effects. Hamid et al. (2015) found that the effect of inositol is enhanced with the addition of d-chiroinositol in a 40:1 ratio, and surpasses the benefits of metformin in terms of weight reduction, resumption of spontaneous ovulation, and spontaneous pregnancy. In the first comparison of metformin and inositol, Fruzzetti et al. (2017) (echoed by the results of Nas and Tűű 2017 soon afterwards), found that both had equally good impact of insulin sensitisation; however, the side effects of metformin in 10% of patients—nausea, lack of appetite, and diarrhoea—was bad enough that they risked dropping out of the study.

There is a problem for surgeons in that metformin must not be taken for at least two days prior to surgery due to the risk of metabolic acidosis. There is the added problem for researchers that because metformin is approved for type 2 diabetes, but not for PCOS, extra administration is needed in studies of metformin for PCOS. This problem of prescribing metformin 'off-label' is one that has been noted by researchers (e.g. Muth et al. 2004). Thus, despite the benefits of metformin, the down sides might make it seem less appealing than inositol.

So, why is inositol not being prescribed to women with PCOS at least as often as metformin? Although Fruzzetti et al. (2017) suggest this may be due to the (currently) higher cost of inositol, others urge that we simply need to be very cautious about approving new medications. For example, The Association of UK dieticians (BDA) state that there is 'insufficient evidence to support recommending D-chiro-inositol or myo-inositol for women with PCOS' (Jeanes 2017).

Conclusion

The relationship between testosterone and insulin is a fascinating and complex one. In some ways, we might say that insulin resistance is at the root of PCOS; this way of seeing PCOS takes us one step back from the more immediate problems of hyperandrogenism, and might also help to identify wider solutions.

References

Altuntas, Y., Bilir, M., Ucak, S., & Gundogdu, S. (2005). Reactive hypoglycemia in lean young women with PCOS and correlations with insulin sensitivity and with beta cell function. *European Journal of Obstetrics & Gynecology and Reproductive Biology, 119*, 198–205.

Asik, M., Altinbas, K., Eroglu, M., Karaahmet, E., Erbag, G., Ertekin, H., & Sen, H. (2015). Evaluation of affective temperament and anxiety–depression levels of patients with polycystic ovary syndrome. *Journal of Affective Disorders, 185*, 214–218.

Azziz, R., Carmina, E., Dewailly, D., Diamanti-Kandarakis, E., Escobar-Morreale, H. F., Futterweit, W., … (Task Force on the Phenotype of the Polycystic Ovary Syndrome of The Androgen Excess and PCOS Society). (2008). The Androgen Excess and PCOS Society criteria for the polycystic ovary syndrome: The complete task force report. *Fertility and Sterility, 91*, 456–488.

Barry, J. A., Hardiman, P. J., Saxby, B. K., & Kuczmierczyk, A. (2011b). Testosterone and mood dysfunction in women with polycystic ovarian syndrome compared to subfertile controls. *Journal of Psychosomatic Obstetrics and Gynecology, 32*(2), 104–111.

Barry, J. A., Bouloux, P., & Hardiman, P. J. (2011c). The impact of eating behavior on psychological symptoms typical of reactive hypoglycemia. A pilot study comparing women with polycystic ovary syndrome to controls. *Appetite, 57*(1), 73–76.

Bartholome, L. T., Raymond, N. C., Lee, S. S., Peterson, C. B., & Warren, C. S. (2006). Detailed analysis of binges in obese women with binge eating disorder: Comparisons using multiple methods of data collection. *International Journal of Eating Disorders, 39*(8), 685–693.

Batool, S., ul ain Ahmed, F., Ambreen, A., Sheikh, A., & Faryad, N. (2016). Depression and anxiety in women with polycystic ovary syndrome and its biochemical associates. *Journal of South Asian Federation of Obstetrics and Gynaecology, 8*(1), 44–47.

Bellver, J., Rodriguez-Tabernero, L., Robles, A., Muñoz, E., Martínez, F., Landeras, J., … Acevedo, B. (2018). Polycystic ovary syndrome throughout a woman's life. *Journal of Assisted Reproduction and Genetics, 35*(1), 25–39.

Brand-Miller, J., Farid, N. R., & Marsh, K. (2004). *The low GI guide to managing PCOS*. London: Hodder & Stoughton.

Buffington, C. K., Kitabchi, A. E., & Givens, J. R. (1991). Adiposity, hyperandrogenism, and hyperinsulinemia in females. *In Program of the Endocrine Society.*

Burghen, G. A., Givens, J. R., & Kitabchi, A. E. (1980). Correlation of hyperandrogenism with hyperinsulinism in polycystic ovarian disease. *The Journal of Clinical Endocrinology and Metabolism, 50,* 113–116.

Cesta, C. E., Månsson, M., Palm, C., Lichtenstein, P., Iliadou, A. N., & Landén, M. (2016). Polycystic ovary syndrome and psychiatric disorders: Co-morbidity and heritability in a nationwide Swedish cohort. *Psychoneuroendocrinology, 73,* 196–203.

Cinar, N., Kizilarslanoglu, M. C., Harmanci, A., Aksoy, D. Y., Bozdag, G., Demir, B., & Yildiz, B. O. (2011). Depression, anxiety and cardiometabolic risk in polycystic ovary syndrome. *Human Reproduction, 26,* 3339–3345.

Diamanti-Kandarakis, E., & Christakou, C. D. (2009). Insulin resistance in PCOS. In *Diagnosis and management of polycystic ovary syndrome* (pp. 35–61). Boston, MA: Springer.

Diamanti-Kandarakis, E., & Papavassiliou, A. G. (2006). Molecular mechanisms of insulin resistance in polycystic ovary syndrome. *Trends in Molecular Medicine, 12*(7), 324–332.

Diamanti-Kandarakis, E., Argyrakopoulou, G., Economou, F., Kandaraki, E., & Koutsilieris, M. (2008). Defects in insulin signaling pathways in ovarian steroidogenesis and other tissues in polycystic ovary syndrome (PCOS). *The Journal of Steroid Biochemistry and Molecular Biology, 109*(3–5), 242–246.

Diamanti-Kandarakis, E., Mitrakou, A., Hennes, M. M., Platanissiotis, D., Kaklas, N., Spina, J., … Raptis, S. (1995). Insulin sensitivity and antiandrogenic therapy in women with polycystic ovary syndrome. *Metabolism, Clinical and Experimental, 44,* 525–531.

Ding, T., Hardiman, P. J., Petersen, I., & Baio, G. (2018). Incidence and prevalence of diabetes and cost of illness analysis of polycystic ovary syndrome: A Bayesian modelling study. *Human Reproduction, 33*(7), 1299–1306.

Dunaif, A., & Book, C. B. (1997). Insulin resistance in the polycystic ovary syndrome. In *Clinical research in diabetes and obesity* (pp. 249–274). Totowa, NJ: Humana Press.

Dunaif, A., Segal, K. R., Futterweit, W., & Dobrjansky, A. (1989). Profound peripheral insulin resistance, independent of obesity, in polycystic ovary syndrome. *Diabetes, 38,* 1165–1174.

Enjezab, B., Eftekhar, M., & Mohajeri, M. (2015). Depression and clinical markers in polycystic ovary syndrome. *Iranian Journal of Reproductive Medicine.*

Erensoy, H., Niafar, M., Ghafarzadeh, S., Aghamohammadzadeh, N., & Nader, N. D. (2019). A pilot trial of metformin for insulin resistance and mood disturbances in adolescent and adult women with polycystic ovary syndrome. *Gynecological Endocrinology, 35*(1), 72–75.

Fairburn, C. G., Cooper, Z., & O'connor, M. E. (2008). Eating disorder examination (Edition 16.0D). In N. Y. Guilford Press & C. G. Fairburn (Eds.), *Cognitive behavior therapy and eating disorders* (pp. 265–308). New York: Guilford Press.

Farrell, K., & Antoni, M. H. (2010). Insulin resistance, obesity, inflammation, and depression in polycystic ovary syndrome: Biobehavioral mechanisms and interventions. *Fertility and Sterility, 94*(5), 1565–1574.

First, M. B., Gibbon, M., Spitzer, R. L., & Williams, J. B. W. (1996). *Users guide for the structured clinical interview for DSM IV axis I disorders—Research version (SCID-I, version 2.0)*. New York: New York State Psychiatric Institute.

Fruzzetti, F., Perini, D., Russo, M., Bucci, F., & Gadducci, A. (2017). Comparison of two insulin sensitizers, metformin and myo-inositol, in women with polycystic ovary syndrome (PCOS). *Gynecological Endocrinology, 33*(1), 39–42.

Garner, D. M., Olmsted, M. P., Bohr, Y., & Garfinkel, P. E. (1982). The eating attitudes test: Psychometric features and clinical correlates. *Psychological Medicine, 12*(4), 871–878.

Greenwood, E. A., Pasch, L. A., Shinkai, K., Cedars, M. I., & Huddleston, H. G. (2015). Putative role for insulin resistance in depression risk in polycystic ovary syndrome. *Fertility and Sterility, 104*(3), 707–714.

Greenwood, E. A., Pasch, L. A., Cedars, M. I., Legro, R. S., Huddleston, H. G., & Network, H. D. R. M., & Eunice Kennedy Shriver National Institute of Child Health. (2018). Association among depression, symptom experience, and quality of life in polycystic ovary syndrome. *American Journal of Obstetrics and Gynecology, 219*(3), 279–2e1.

Hamid, A. M. S. A., Madkour, W. A. I., & Borg, T. F. (2015). Inositol versus Metformin administration in polycystic ovary syndrome patients: A case–control study. *Journal of Evidence-Based Women's Health Journal Society, 5*(3), 93–98.

Himelein, M. J., & Thatcher, S. S. (2006). Depression and body image among women with polycystic ovary syndrome. *Journal of Health Psychology, 11*(4), 613–625.

Hirschberg, A., Naessen, S., Stridsberg, M., Byström, B., & Holte, J. (2004). Impaired cholecystokinin secretion and disturbed appetite regulation in women with polycystic ovary syndrome. *Gynecological Endocrinology, 19*(2), 79–87.

Hollinrake, E., Abreu, A., Maifeld, M., Van Voorhis, B. J., & Dokras, A. (2007). Increased risk of depressive disorders in women with polycystic ovary syndrome. *Fertility and Sterility, 87,* 1369–1376.

Hunter, M. H., & Sterrett, J. J. (2000). Polycystic ovary syndrome: It's not just infertility. *American Family Physician, 62,* 1079–1088.

Iwasa, T., Matsuzaki, T., Yano, K., Yiliyasi, M., Kuwahara, A., Matsui, S., & Irahara, M. (2018). Effects of chronic testosterone administration on the degree of preference for a high-fat diet and body weight in gonadal-intact and ovariectomized female rats. *Behavioural Brain Research, 349,* 102–108.

Jaliseh, H. K., Tehrani, F. R., Behboudi-Gandevani, S., Hosseinpanah, F., Khalili, D., Cheraghi, L., & Azizi, F. (2017). Polycystic ovary syndrome is a risk factor for diabetes and prediabetes in middle-aged but not elderly women: A long-term population-based follow-up study. *Fertility and Sterility, 108*(6), 1078–1084.

Jeanes, Y. M., Reeves, S., Gibson, E. L., Piggott, C., May, V. A., & Hart, K. H. (2017). Binge eating behaviours and food cravings in women with polycystic ovary syndrome. *Appetite, 109,* 24–32.

Karacan, E., Caglar, G. S., Gürsoy, A. Y., & Yilmaz, M. B. (2014). Body satisfaction and eating attitudes among girls and young women with and without polycystic ovary syndrome. *Journal of Pediatric and Adolescent Gynecology, 27*(2), 72–77.

Kasim-Karakas, S. E., Cunningham, W. M., & Tsodikov, A. (2007). Relation of nutrients and hormones in polycystic ovary syndrome. *American Journal of Clinical Nutrition, 85,* 688–694.

Kerchner, A., Lester, W., Stuart, S. P., & Dokras, A. (2009). Risk of depression and other mental health disorders in women with polycystic ovary syndrome: A longitudinal study. *Fertility and Sterility, 91*(1), 207–212.

Kissebah, A. H., Freedman, D. S., & Peiris, A. N. (1989). Health risks of obesity. *Medical Clinics of North America, 73*(1), 111–138.

Larsson, I., Hulthén, L., Landén, M., Pålsson, E., Janson, P., & Stener-Victorin, E. (2016). Dietary intake, resting energy expenditure, and eating behavior in women with and without polycystic ovary syndrome. *Clinical Nutrition, 35*(1), 213–218.

Lee, I., Cooney, L. G., Saini, S., Smith, M. E., Sammel, M. D., Allison, K. C., & Dokras, A. (2017). Increased risk of disordered eating in polycystic ovary syndrome. *Fertility and Sterility, 107*(3), 796–802.

Lee, I., Cooney, L. G., Saini, S., Sammel, M. D., Allison, K. C., & Dokras, A. (2018). Increased odds of disordered eating in polycystic ovary syndrome: A systematic review and meta-analysis. *Eating and Weight Disorders—Studies on Anorexia, Bulimia and Obesity.* https://doi.org/10.1007/s40519-018-0533-y

Maharaj, S., & Amod, A. (2009). Polycystic ovary syndrome. *Journal of Endocrinology, Metabolism and Diabetes of South Africa, 14*(2), 86–95.

Månsson, M., Holte, J., Landin-Wilhelmsen, K., Dahlgren, E., Johansson, A., & Landén, M. (2008). Women with polycystic ovary syndrome are often depressed or anxious—A case control study. *Psychoneuroendocrinology, 33*(8), 1132–1138.

Mantantzis, K., Schlaghecken, F., Sünram-Lea, S. I., & Maylor, E. A. (2019). Sugar rush or sugar crash? A meta-analysis of carbohydrate effects on mood. *Neuroscience & Biobehavioral Reviews.*

Marsh, K. A., Steinbeck, K. S., Atkinson, F. S., Petocz, P., & Brand-Miller, J. C. (2010). Effect of a low glycemic index compared with a conventional healthy diet on polycystic ovary syndrome. *The American Journal of Clinical Nutrition, 92*(1), 83–92.

Moghetti, P., Castello, R., Negri, C., Tosi, F., Perrone, F., Caputo, M., … Muggeo, M. (2000). Metformin effects on clinical features, endocrine and metabolic profiles, and insulin sensitivity in polycystic ovary syndrome: A randomized, double-blind, placebo-controlled 6-month trial, followed by open, long-term clinical evaluation. *The Journal of Clinical Endocrinology & Metabolism, 85*(1), 139–146.

Moran, L. J., Misso, M. L., Wild, R. A., & Norman, R. J. (2010). Impaired glucose tolerance, type 2 diabetes and metabolic syndrome in polycystic ovary syndrome: A systematic review and meta-analysis. *Human Reproduction Update, 16*(4), 347–363.

Morgan, J. F., McCluskey, S. E., Brunton, J. N., & Lacey, J. H. (2002). Polycystic ovarian morphology and bulimia nervosa: A 9-year follow-up study. *Fertility and Sterility, 77*(5), 928–931.

Muth, S., Norman, J., Sattar, N., & Fleming, R. (2004). Women with polycystic ovary syndrome (PCOS) often undergo protracted treatment with metformin and are disinclined to stop: Indications for a change in licensing arrangements? *Human Reproduction, 19*(12), 2718–2720.

Nas, K., & Tűű, L. (2017). A comparative study between myo-inositol and metformin in the treatment of insulin-resistant women. *European Review for Medical and Pharmacological Sciences, 21*(2 Suppl), 77–82.

Nestler, J. E., Powers, L. P., Matt, D. W., Steingold, K. A., Plymate, S. R., Rittmaster, R. S., ... Blackard, W. G. (1991). A direct effect of hyperinsulinemia on serum sex hormone binding globulin levels in obese women with the polycystic ovary syndrome. *The Journal of Clinical Endocrinology and Metabolism, 72*, 83–89.

NHS. (2017). Binge eating disorder. Retrieved May 21, 2019, from https://www.nhs.uk/conditions/binge-eating/.

Norman, R., Wu, R., & Stankiewicz, M. (2004). Polycystic ovary syndrome. *The Medical Journal of Australia, 180*(3), 132–137.

Ovalle, F., & Azziz, R. (2002). Insulin resistance, polycystic ovary syndrome, and type 2 diabetes mellitus. *Fertility and Sterility, 77*(6), 1095–1105.

Ozdemir, O., Kurdoğlu, Z., Yıldız, S., Özdemir, P. G., & Yilmaz, E. (2016). The relationship between atypical depression and insülin resistance in patients with polycystic ovary syndrome and major depression. *Psychiatry Research*.

Paganini, C., Peterson, G., Stavropoulos, V., & Krug, I. (2018). The overlap between binge eating behaviors and polycystic ovarian syndrome: An etiological integrative model. *Current Pharmaceutical Design, 24*(9), 999–1006.

Parry, S., Woods, R., Hodson, L., & Hulston, C. (2017). A single day of excessive dietary fat intake reduces whole-body insulin sensitivity: The metabolic consequence of binge eating. *Nutrients, 9*(8), 818.

Pasquali, R., Gambineri, A., Biscotti, D., Vicennati, V., Gagliardi, L., Colitta, D., ... Morselli-Labate, A. M. (2000). Effect of long-term treatment with metformin added to hypocaloric diet on body composition, fat distribution, and androgen and insulin levels in abdominally obese women with and without the polycystic ovary syndrome. *The Journal of Clinical Endocrinology & Metabolism, 85*(8), 2767–2774.

Rasgon, N. L., Carter, M. S., Elman, S., Bauer, M., Love, M., & Korenman, S. G. (2002). Common treatment of polycystic ovarian syndrome and major depressive disorder: Case report and review. *Current Drug Targets-Immune, Endocrine & Metabolic Disorders, 2*(1), 97–102.

Sam, S. (2007). Obesity and polycystic ovary syndrome. *Obesity Management, 3*, 69–73.

Sørensen, M., & Johansen, O. E. (2010). Idiopathic reactive hypoglycaemia—Prevalence and effect of fibre on glucose excursions. *Scandinavian Journal of Clinical and Laboratory Investigation, 70*, 385–391.

Stanley, T., & Misra, M. (2008). Polycystic ovary syndrome in obese adolescents. *Current Opinion in Endocrinology, Diabetes, and Obesity, 15*, 30–36.

Stice, E., & Shaw, H. E. (2002). Role of body dissatisfaction in the onset and maintenance of eating pathology: A synthesis of research findings. *Journal of Psychosomatic Research, 53*(5), 985–993.

Sundblad, C., Bergman, L., & Eriksson, E. (1994). High levels of free testosterone in women with bulimia nervosa. *Acta Psychiatrica Scandinavica, 90*(5), 397–398.

Sundblad, C., Landén, M., Eriksson, T., Bergman, L., & Eriksson, E. (2005). Effects of the androgen antagonist flutamide and the serotonin reuptake inhibitor citalopram in bulimia nervosa: A placebo-controlled pilot study. *Journal of Clinical Psychopharmacology, 25*(1), 85–88.

Taylor, A. E., Hubbard, J., & Anderson, E. J. (1999). Impact of binge eating on metabolic and leptin dynamics in normal young women. *The Journal of Clinical Endocrinology and Metabolism, 84*(2), 428–434.

Thayer, R. E. (1987). Energy, tiredness, and tension effects of a sugar snack versus moderate exercise. *Journal of Personality and Social Psychology, 52*(1), 119.

Unfer, V., Carlomagno, G., Dante, G., & Facchinetti, F. (2012). Effects of myoinositol in women with PCOS: A systematic review of randomized controlled trials. *Gynecological Endocrinology, 28*(7), 509–515.

Yen, S. S. C. (1991). Chronic anovulation caused by peripheral report. J. Clin. Psychiatry 61, 173–178. endocrine disorders. In S. S. C. Yen & R. B. Jaffe (Eds.), *Reproductive endocrinology: physiology, pathophysiology and clin. Management* (3rd ed., pp. 576–630). Philadelphia: W.B. Saunders.

Zhao, Y., & Qiao, J. (2013). Ethnic differences in the phenotypic expression of polycystic ovary syndrome. *Steroids, 78*(8), 755–760.

6

Fertility and Psychology in PCOS

Abstract It is popularly thought that stress can have a negative impact on fertility, but what is the evidence for this? In this chapter, the ways in which psychology and biology can interact to impact fertility are described. This chapter also assesses the impact of PCOS on sexual functioning and satisfaction, and explores evidence for how oral contraceptives—often prescribed in PCOS—might impact psychological functioning.

Keywords Fertility • Psychoneuroimmunology • Sexual functioning • Sexual satisfaction • Oral contraceptive

Introduction

Infertility is clinically defined as being unable to conceive within 12 months (Abma 1997). In the general population, about a third of infertility is cause by male issues, about a third by female. Of the remaining third about half is some combination of male and female issues, and about half is unexplained (American Society for Reproductive Medicine (ASRM 2019)). The most common cause of infertility in women is anovulatory PCOS. Around 40% of women with PCOS experience

© The Author(s) 2019
J. A. Barry, *Psychological Aspects of Polycystic Ovary Syndrome*,
https://doi.org/10.1007/978-3-030-30290-0_6

infertility, and the cause is infrequent or absent ovulation (Jayasena and Franks 2014). Various other factors have been implicated for infertility in PCOS, but by far the clearest evidence is for the role of insufficient serum FSH. Also, fertility problems are exacerbated in PCOS because elevated testosterone and BMI disrupt the menstrual cycle.

The ASRM states that 'Infertility often creates one of the most distressing life crises that a couple has ever experienced together' (ASRM 2019). A review of quality of life (QoL) issues in the general population found that women with fertility problems tended to have worse QoL than healthy women, and worse QoL health than men with fertility problems (Chachamovich et al. 2010). It should be noted however that this review excluded PCOS and other conditions (e.g. endometriosis and cancer) for which infertility is a secondary consequence. Also, most participants were recruited from fertility clinics, thus possibly more distressed than infertile women not seeking fertility treatment. Although the evidence in PCOS research is a little more mixed, it seems likely that fertility problems impact women with PCOS to a similar degree to non-PCOS women who experience fertility problems (Barry et al. 2011). Women with PCOS have the added impact of the other distressing symptoms of PCOS (Barry et al. 2018).

This chapter will focus on the impact of infertility on levels of distress. It will also explore evidence that causality can work in the opposite direction, that is, distress can impact levels of fertility. The chapter will also explore sexual functioning and satisfaction in PCOS, treatments for infertility in PCOS, and address the question of how much impact there is of oral contraceptives on psychological functioning. Some of the research discussed here is based on findings from non-PCOS research, so appropriate allowances for poorly fitting generalisations to women with PCOS should be applied to that research.

Depression, QoL, and Infertility in PCOS

Most studies of fertility problems in PCOS find an association with distress. Bazarganipour et al. (2013) assessed 300 women with PCOS in Iran and found that infertile women had significantly lower levels of self-esteem and body satisfaction. Trent (2003) found that adolescents with PCOS were 3.4 times more likely than healthy controls to have worries about future fertility. In a study of 40 Polish women with PCOS aged 20–30 years, it was found they were more anxious than 40 menopausal women, and than 20 women post mastectomy (Mącik 2016). Their anxiety was centred around uncertainty about fertility outcomes.

McCook et al. (2005) found that women with PCOS who had miscarried had lower PCOSQ scores than women with PCOS who had not ever succeeded in becoming pregnant. van Wely et al. (2004) found that successful treatment of infertility improved QoL in women with PCOS. Despite a small sample size, Deeks et al. (2010) found statistically significantly higher rates of HADS depression in 23 infertile women with PCOS compared to 25 women with PCOS who were fertile. The infertile women scored higher on several other measures of distress, but these differences did not reach statistical significance, due to the small sample size reducing the power of the statistical tests to identify group differences.

However, not all studies have found an effect of infertility on women with PCOS. For example, McCook (2002) and Himelein and Thatcher (2006) found no significant difference between the depression ratings of fertile and infertile women with PCOS. Tan et al. (2008) assessed the psychological impact of infertility in 115 women with PCOS, comparing their scores on various psychometric tests to normative scores. Although 51% of the women had a current wish to conceive and 76% worried about being childless in the future, the authors report that this did not impact depressive symptoms, quality-of-life, or emotional distress. However, closer inspection of the findings suggests that this interpretation of the data may be due to methodological issues. Firstly, the sample size (n = 115) will have underpowered the Chi Square test, meaning that any differences between groups will be less likely to be identified as statistically significant. Also, there was the reduction of statistical significance by using the Bonferroni correction, a statistical adjustment that should be used with caution, especially when assessing relatively under-researched areas, such as the impact of infertility on women with PCOS. Interestingly, they found that the rate of depression in women with an unfulfilled wish to conceive was higher in the 'mild to moderate depression' category (28.3% vs 22.4%), but lower in the 'clinical depression' category (20.8% vs 28.6%). To some degree this explains the puzzling finding that women with an unfulfilled wish to conceive had, on average, lower depression scores than those without such wishes (11.7 ± 9.2 vs 14.25 ± 11.1), so part of the explanation of this finding is that group means were skewed by some of the women with no unfulfilled wish to conceive being relatively severely depressed. Why might that be so? A clue might be in the differences in demographics of each group: the group who didn't want to conceive were significantly younger (26.7 vs 29.4 years old), were significantly more likely to be single (93% vs 54%), and were more likely to have children (16% vs 7%). It could be that the fact of being a mother means that these women didn't have an unfulfilled wish to conceive, and being a young single mother makes for a difficult life. The methodological issues of this study mean that we can draw no firm conclusions from it about the impact of fertility on the psychology of women with PCOS. Apart from the issues already mentioned, it is also in doubt that the distributions were non-normal in the BDI scores, meaning that the Mann-Whitney test might have been a preferred alternative to the t-test. However the main weakness of this study was that relevant group differences were not controlled for.

The Impact of Distress on Fertility in Women in General

At present, there is no research on the impact of stress in PCOS on fertility, so note that this section is about the general population.

Fertility problems are known to cause distress (e.g. Deeks et al. 2010), but it is important to note that the causality may be reciprocal, that is, there is evidence that psychological stress can impair fertility (Boivin and Takefman 1995). Evidence for this effect comes in various forms. For example, a meta-analysis Qu et al. (2017) found that risk of miscarriage was significantly higher in women with a history of exposure to psychological stress. A study of 742 women in the US found that, independent of age, BMI, race, education, smoking, and income, the greater the number of adverse childhood events, the greater the degree of fertility difficulties and amenorrhea (Jacobs et al. 2015).

How can distress impact fertility? Well, in his classic studies, Selye (1950) found that exposure to stressors caused ovarian atrophy in rats. Psychological anxiety can activate the HPA axis, and because stress hormones interact with fertility hormones such as LH (luetinising hormone) and FSH (follicle-stimulating hormone), this means that the HPG (hypothalamic-pituitary gonadal) axis is also vulnerable to the effects of stress (Berga 1996). Rivest and Rivier (1995) found that cortisol reduces levels of sex hormones by disrupting their synthesis. Anxiety and high cortisol levels, depression, avoidance and high expression of emotion have been associated with lower pregnancy rates after fertility treatment (Demyttenaere et al. 1992; Smeenk et al. 2001, 2005). Smeenk et al. (2001) found that anxiety and to a lesser extent depression were significantly negatively correlated with pregnancy outcome in their study of 291 women who underwent fertility treatment with IVF/ICSI (in vitro fertilisation/intracytoplasmic sperm injection). Klonoff-Cohen et al. (2001) suggest that while the anxiety generated by fertility treatment procedures affects biological outcomes (for example, number of oocytes fertilised), baseline measures of acute and chronic stress are related to pregnancy outcomes such as birth weight.

Cesta (2017) studied a large register of Swedish women in the general population. They found that of the 23,557 women undergoing an IVF cycle, the 164 with a depression/anxiety diagnosis (probably relatively severe) prior to pregnancy who did not take an antidepressant had a reduced chance of pregnancy (adjusted OR = 0.58) and reduced change of live birth (adjusted OR = 0.60). This effect was less in the 829 women who had been taking an SSRI (selective serotonin reuptake inhibitor, such as Prozac).

Cwikel et al. (2004) suggest that chronic stress should be treated prior to fertility treatment, and although there has been very little research in this area there is evidence that psychological interventions improve fertility rates. For example, a small study by Sarrel and DeCherney (1985) found that a psychotherapeutic interview yielded a pregnancy rate of 60% for 10 infertile couples compared to 10% for 10 controls. In a small

RCT, Hosaka et al. (2002) found that 37 women receiving five weekly 90-minute sessions of relaxation, guided imagery, and stress management had reduced emotional distress and improved the pregnancy rate compared to 37 controls (38% vs 14%). Natural Killer (NK) cell activity was also lower in the treatment group (48% vs 34%). NK cell activity is not usually measured in fertility studies, but high NK cell activity has been observed in idiopathic infertile women and unexplained recurrent miscarriage (Matsubayashi et al. 2005). Levitas et al. (2006) used a single session of hypnosis with 89 patients during the embryo transfer procedure and found a significantly higher pregnancy rate than 96 no-hypnosis controls (58% vs 30%, $p < 0.05$). The hypnosis group also had a higher implantation rate (28% vs 14%, $p < 0.001$). Domar (2000), however, found no significant effect of CBT + relaxation on pregnancy outcomes in a randomised controlled trial (RCT) of 184 women.

There is some evidence in non-PCOS populations that having children in later life is impacted by personality and perhaps early childhood experiences. For example, Hadley et al. (2019) found that independent of other variables (age, sex, medical issues, education level, marital status, recent life stress, health-related quality of life, mental positivity, and avoidant attachment style), men and women who were childless by age 50 or older were significantly more likely to have developed an anxious attachment to their primary caregiver in childhood. It is known that that adults with signs of childhood attachment issues report lower relationship satisfaction (Barry et al. 2015), and it could be that women with PCOS—who are more likely to be socially avoidant (as discussed in Chap. 3) possibly due to having embarrassing symptoms—might have even more difficultly forming relationships and having children if they have had formed an anxious childhood attachment.

As is seen with the QoL measures (Chap. 3), self-reported anxiety is not always reflected in objective measures (for example Gold et al. 2003), which might impact research on the influence of distress on fertility. There is also the methodological issue of establishing the amount of variance in anxiety ratings that could be a cause (trait/chronic anxiety) or result (state anxiety) of fertility issues; this is a complex task, not least because the relationship between infertility and psychological problems is probably reciprocal.

Sexual Functioning and Satisfaction in Women with PCOS

The evidence in this field is somewhat mixed. Reflecting this, a meta-analysis of 19 studies (Murgel et al. 2019) found no real impact of PCOS on sexual function and satisfaction. However overall it seems that women with PCOS may experience doubts about their sexual attractiveness, causing discomfort or disinterest when it comes to sex. Another meta-analysis (Pastoor et al. 2018) highlighted significant small detriments in PCOS compared to other women for sexual arousal, lubrication, sexual satisfaction, and orgasm.

Although Pastoor et al. found that body hair and body image had an impact on sex, the impact of body weight was not specifically assessed. Stapinska-Syniec et al. (2018) assessed 250 women with PCOS and found that overweight women felt less attractive, and less attractive women reported less sexual satisfaction. Stovall et al. (2012) found that high BMI was associated with a significant reduction of orgasm. Morotti et al. (2013) found no significant difference in self-esteem, body image, depression levels, and sexual functioning between 33 lean women with PCOS and 22 healthy women, despite the moderate hirsutism and hyperandrogenism in the PCOS group. The findings of Morotti et al. imply that BMI is relevant to sexual functioning in non-lean women with PCOS, but not all studies find this link: neither de Niet et al. (2012) nor Benetti-Pinto et al. (2015) found that BMI is correlated with sexual function in PCOS. The possible impact of BMI on sexual functioning is a topic worth further investigation.

Stovall et al. (2012) found no reduction in sexual desire and orgasms in 92 women with PCOS compared with 82 controls. Bazarganipour et al. (2014) used structural equation modelling to analyse data from 300 women with PCOS in Iran. They found that the clinical aspects of PCOS impacted self-esteem, body image, and with regard to sexual functioning, impacted desire and arousal. However, they did not compare the findings of the PCOS group to a control group of any kind, making their findings less informative. Zueff et al. (2015) found that PCOS was not a predictor of sexual functioning, but the logistic regression they used was underpowered by the small sample size (87 women in total, and 9 predictor variables).

Intuitively (and based on evidence in Chap. 4), we would expect that higher testosterone would lead to higher libido. In keeping with these expectations, Stovall et al. (2012) noted that women with the highest testosterone levels had also significantly better sexual functioning. Controlling for other variables, Amiri et al. (2018) found that among 492 women with PCOS, there was a correlation between testosterone and libido. Also they found a correlation between increased sexual function and FAI, but only in those with the highest FAI levels (>4.5 nmol/L), and then, the correlation was not statistically significant. In contrast, Rellini et al. (2013) found hyperandrogenic women had lower sexual desire, and Ercan et al. (2013) found a negative correlation between androgen and sexual functioning. Other authors have found no link between libido and testosterone in PCOS (McCook 2002; Conaglen and Conaglen 2003; de Niet et al. 2012).

In a study of 480 women with PCOS, de Niet et al. (2012) found that hirsute women with PCOS were older than non-hirsute women with PCOS when they had their first romantic relationship, and were less likely to have been in love more than once. It is worth noting that despite the impact of PCOS sexual desire, McCook (2002) found that relationship satisfaction was not impacted.

Psychological Impact of Oral Contraceptives for PCOS

A few words should be said about the impact of oral contraceptive use in PCOS. Like metformin, they are commonly prescribed for PCOS though remain 'off-label' because they are not specifically licenced for this use. One of the treatment strategies for PCOS is the combined oral contraceptive pill (OCP). The most commonly prescribed in PCOS are Co-cyprindiol (marketed as *Dianette*) and ethinyl estradiol/drospirenone (*Yasmin*). Sometimes women are puzzled that they are being given a contraceptive when they are not wishing to prevent pregnancy, but there is a reason for their use in PCOS. These pills are 'combined' because they: (a) contain progestogen which, by LH suppression, prevents the ovaries from producing androgen, and (b) contain estrogen, which increases SHGB levels, which reduces the amount of active androgen. Some combined pills also contain an anti-androgen, such as cyproterone acetate in Dianette, or drospirenone in Yasmin. Dianette and Yasmin thus have a slight advantage over other combined pills for women with PCOS, with mild to moderate improvements seen in acne and hirsutism within 3–6 months (Graham and Hamoda 2016). Furthermore, they can also help protect against endometrial cancer, a cancer for which women with PCOS are at increased risk (Anderson et al. 2014).

Although some years ago, Dianette was reviewed by the health authorities over concerns of it causing depression, the National Institute for Health and Care Excellence (NICE) today lists the risk of depression only under 'Cautions' as an issue for 'women with a history of severe depression especially if induced by hormonal contraceptive', and as a side effect, the risk of depression is listed under 'Frequency not known' (NICE 2019b). However, although fears regarding Dianette causing depression are reduced, it is recognised that Dianette increases the risk of venous thromboembolism (blood clotting).

There is some interesting literature on the psychological impact of using 'the pill', as oral contraceptives are popularly known, although the literature is not always clear on which type of contraceptive is being referred to, so not all of the research findings generalise to women with PCOS, who are generally prescribed either Dianette or Yasmin. A further complication is indicated by a review of hormonal contraceptives which found that evidence from RCTs suggest that most of the side effects experienced by women are psychological responses to the practice of contraception, rather than responses to hormonal disruption (Robinson et al. 2004). There is also the question of whether the contractive pill contributes to the problem of endocrine disruptors in the environment (see Chap. 1). This is because the estrogenic capacity of the pill is not broken down in the body, and is excreted from the body, where it remains bioactive in the environment (Owen and Jobling 2012).

Fortunately, there have also a few studies of oral contraceptive use in PCOS. Possibly more would have been done on this topic, but it is often difficult to get approval for research of this kind because OCPs are not specifically licenced for use in PCOS. Cinar et al. (2012) conducted a study of the impact of Yasmin on QoL and mood outcomes over a period of 6 months with 36 women with PCOS in Turkey. Although testosterone, the free androgen index, DHEAS, and hirsutism (measured using the Ferriman-Gallwey assessment) significantly improved over the study period—as did PCOSQ scores for emotions, body hair, and infertility—HADS and BDI remained unchanged. In an online study, Barnard et al. (2007) found mixed evidence regarding the benefits of anti-androgen medication for women with PCOS. There was no consistent difference in depression scores or PCOSQ scores between women with PCOS taking anti-androgen medication compared to those not taking anti-androgen medication. However the validity of this Barnard et al. finding is in question because it included a wide variety of medications in the category of anti-androgens: metformin, various oral contraceptives, contraceptive implants and injections, and the herbal remedy *agnus castus*, typically used to treat PMS. In a much more methodologically robust study, Dokras et al. (2016) conducted an RCT of overweight/obese women with PCOS, randomising 132 women to 16 weeks of either oral contraceptive or lifestyle modification (diet, exercise, and weight loss medication), or both interventions combined. They found in the OCP group depression prevalence decreased significantly from 13.3% to 4.4% ($p < 0.05$), and anxiety improved non-significantly. PCOSQ scores improved in all three groups.

Treatment for Infertility in PCOS

There is some evidence that when the problems related to PCOS are reduced, this has a beneficial impact on QoL. For example, van Wely et al. (2004) randomised 168 women with PCOS into two fertility treatment conditions (laparoscopic electrocautery vs recombinant follicle-stimulating hormone) and found that successful fertility treatment improved Short Form 36 (SF-36) scores (a measure of HRQoL) for emotional and mental health problems, though also increased role limitations (for example, feeling that they had accomplished less) due to normal physical restrictions of pregnancy.

We might expect that one of the biggest improvements to QoL for a subfertile woman is to become fertile and have a baby. Although there has not been a great deal of research on this topic, it is worth having a brief review of some of the fertility treatments that are available. Note that this is not a comprehensive review, and interested readers should look at the original sources cited for further information.

Anovulation in PCOS is caused by insufficient levels of serum FSH, so interventions tend to be aimed at raising FSH to levels seen in the early follicular phase of the normal menstrual cycle. However because being overweight reduces ovulatory frequency, the first intervention usually suggested is diet and lifestyle changes (Jayasena and Franks 2014). This make sense because a meta-analysis of the impact of maternal obesity on infant outcomes found that when BMI is taken into account, there is no additional risk of PCOS for preterm birth, lower birth weight, higher gestational weight gain, and 'large for gestational age' births (Bahri Khomami et al. 2019).

Metformin is often the next level of intervention. A review of metformin versus placebo studies found improved ovulation and a mean reduction of 0.6 nmol/L in testosterone, but no difference in BMI or miscarriage risk (Tang et al. 2012). However, subsequent research pooling the findings of three large RCTs in Scandinavia found a significant reduction in late miscarriages and preterm births (a composite outcome) in the metformin group (5%) compared to placebo (10%) (Løvvik et al. 2019). This study confirms previous findings that metformin does not significantly reduce gestational diabetes.

If pregnancy hasn't been achieved by other means, six cycles of Clomifene citrate (Clomid) are commonly used to improve ovulation. This is a selective estrogen-receptor modulator (SERM), which induces gonadotropin release by blocking the hypothalamic estrogen receptors, which disrupt hypothalamic-pituitary-ovarian (HPO) axis feedback mechanisms (NICE 2019a). Clomifene treatment has a live birth rate of 23%. However there are risks: multiple ovulation and ovarian hyperstimulation syndrome (OHSS) need to be monitored in the first cycle, multiple pregnancy occurs in 4%–8% of cases, and it can be used for only 6 cycles because of the theoretical risk of ovarian cancer. An alternative to clomifene is Letrozole. This is an aromatase inhibitor and prevents the conversion of testosterone to estrogen, which at first seems counterintuitive because estrogen has an important role in ovulation. However it works because it induces the HPO axis to compensate for the lack of estrogen by restarting ovulation (Ecklund and Usadi 2015). Ecklund and Usadi found letrozole is superior to clomifene because it has improved live birth rates and less risk of multiple ovulation and multiple pregnancy rates when compared with clomifene. A meta-analysis comparing Letrozole to ovarian drilling (i.e. removal of the ovarian cysts, usually by laser) found that both were equally effective in achieving live birth rate in women with PCOS, though there was a statistically significant increase in the pregnancy rate in women taking Letrozole compared to those using ovarian drilling (Yu et al. 2019). Because ovarian drilling is invasive (requiring 'keyhole surgery' via the navel), and because it is more expensive, for many women, Letrozole is the chosen option.

An advantage of inositols over metformin is evidence that inositols may reduce gestational diabetes in PCOS (D'Anna et al. 2012) and non-PCOS women with type 2 diabetes (D'Anna et al. 2013). More research is needed on PCOS pregnancies, but D'Anna et al. (2012) found in a study of women with PCOS that 17.4% of the 46 women on inositol developed gestational diabetes compared to 54% of the 37 women taking metformin. However, in light of promising research discussed in the Chap. 5, it is disappointing that a meta-analysis found inositols don't show sufficient benefit to be recommended as an aid to fertility treatment with IVF/ICSI (Bhide et al. 2019). The authors note that the quality of the 18 studies was not very high overall, so better quality research is needed before a more definite opinion can be made.

Fertility treatment is not always successful, and the live birth rate per treatment cycle is generally around 20% (Sullivan et al. 2013). A meta-analysis by Milazzo et al. (2016) found that successful fertility treatment reduces depression scores, but anxiety and depression increased if assisted reproductive technologies (ART) fail. Although women with PCOS are more likely to have issues with depression (see Chap. 2), some good news is that March et al. (2018) found no statistically significant difference in the rate of postnatal depression in 52 women with PCOS compared to 512 other women. However, those women with PCOS who had suffered a miscarriage or required medical assistance to conceive were at a non-significantly ($p < 0.06$) elevated risk of postnatal depression.

Conclusion

PCOS has been called 'the thief of womanhood' (Kitzinger and Willmott 2002), so much of the evidence discussed in this chapter comes to the unsurprising conclusion that having fertility problems is a stressful aspect of PCOS. However, as a general rule, health professionals should personalise treatment for PCOS and not presume that fertility is at the forefront of each patient's mind (Sullivan 2017). For example, although younger women usually don't want to start a family immediately, as they get older they might change their mind, sometimes quite suddenly. Therefore it's only fair to inform younger women of how to prepare for this change in priorities in order to minimise the chances of a lot of stress and expensive fertility treatment later in life. Delivering such news might be taken as patronising to a 20-year-old, but by the time they reach 30 the patient should already know the reality of their chances of conception, and that they should ideally be of a certain BMI, and so on.

More research is needed on women with PCOS for some of the above issues (e.g. in the section on the impact of stress on fertility), because findings from women who don't have PCOS do not necessarily generalise perfectly to women with PCOS.

References

Abma, J. C. (Ed.). (1997). *Fertility, family planning, and women's health: New data from the 1995 National Survey of Family Growth* (Vol. 19). Hyattsville, MD: National Center for Health Statistics.

American Society for Reproductive Medicine. (2019). *FAQs about infertility*. Retrieved May 6, 2019, from https://www.reproductivefacts.org/faqs/frequently-asked-questions-about-infertility/.

Amiri, F. N., Tehrani, F. R., Esmailzadeh, S., Tohidi, M., Azizi, F., & Basirat, Z. (2018). Sexual function in women with polycystic ovary syndrome and their hormonal and clinical correlations. *International Journal of Impotence Research, 30*(2), 54.

Anderson, S. A., Barry, J. A., & Hardiman, P. J. (2014). Risk of coronary heart disease and risk of stroke in women with polycystic ovary syndrome: A systematic review and meta-analysis. *International Journal of Cardiology, 176*(2), 486–487.

Bahri Khomami, M., Joham, A. E., Boyle, J. A., Piltonen, T., Arora, C., Silagy, M., ... Moran, L. J. (2019). The role of maternal obesity in infant outcomes in polycystic ovary syndrome—A systematic review, meta-analysis, and meta-regression. *Obesity Reviews, 20*(6), 842–858.

Barnard, L., Ferriday, D., Guenther, N., Strauss, B., Balen, A. H., & Dye, L. (2007). Quality of life and psychological well being in polycystic ovary syndrome. *Human Reproduction, 22*, 2279–2286.

Barry, J. A., Hardiman, P. J., Saxby, B. K., & Kuczmierczyk, A. (2011). Testosterone and mood dysfunction in women with polycystic ovarian syndrome compared to subfertile controls. *Journal of Psychosomatic Obstetrics and Gynecology, 32*(2), 104–111.

Barry, J. A., Seager, M., & Brown, B. (2015). Gender differences in the association between attachment style and adulthood relationship satisfaction (brief report). *New Male Studies, 4*(3), 63–74.

Barry, J. A., Qu, F., & Hardiman, P. J. (2018). An exploration of the hypothesis that testosterone is implicated in the psychological functioning of women with polycystic ovary syndrome (PCOS). *Medical Hypotheses, 110*, 42–45.

Bazarganipour, F., Ziaei, S., Montazeri, A., Foroozanfard, F., Kazemnejad, A., & Faghihzadeh, S. (2013). Body image satisfaction and self-esteem status among the patients with polycystic ovary syndrome. *Iranian Journal of Reproductive Medicine, 11*(10), 829.

Bazarganipour, F., Ziaei, S., Montazeri, A., Foroozanfard, F., Kazemnejad, A., & Faghihzadeh, S. (2014). Health-related quality of life in patients with polycystic ovary syndrome (PCOS): A model-based study of predictive factors. *The Journal of Sexual Medicine, 11*(4), 1023–1032.

Benetti-Pinto, C. L., Ferreira, S. R., Antunes, A., & Yela, D. A. (2015). The influence of body weight on sexual function and quality of life in women with polycystic ovary syndrome. *Archives of Gynecology and Obstetrics, 291*(2), 451–455.

Berga, S. L. (1996). Stress and ovarian function. *American Journal of Sports Medicine, 24*, S36–S37.

Bhide, P., Pundir, J., Gudi, A., Shah, A., Homburg, R., & Acharya, G. (2019). The effect of myo-inositol/di-chiro-inositol on markers of ovarian reserve in women with PCOS undergoing IVF/ICSI: A systematic review and meta-analysis. *Acta obstetricia et gynecologica Scandinavica.* https://doi.org/10.1111/aogs.13625

Boivin, J., & Takefman, J. E. (1995). Stress level across stages of in vitro fertilization in subsequently pregnant and nonpregnant women. *Fertility and Sterility, 64*, 802–810.

Cesta, C. E. (2017). *Stress, depression, and other psychiatric disorders: An epidemiological approach to studying the causes and consequences for in vitro fertilization outcome and polycystic ovary syndrome.* Thesis. Retrieved from https://openarchive.ki.se/xmlui/handle/10616/45608.

Chachamovich, J. R., Chachamovich, E., Ezer, H., Fleck, M. P., Knauth, D., & Passos, E. P. (2010). Investigating quality of life and health-related quality of life in infertility: A systematic review. *Journal of Psychosomatic Obstetrics and Gynecology, 31*(2), 101–110.

Cinar, N., Harmanci, A., Demir, B., & Yildiz, B. O. (2012). Effect of an oral contraceptive on emotional distress, anxiety and depression of women with polycystic ovary syndrome: A prospective study. *Human Reproduction, 27*(6), 1840–1845.

Conaglen, H. M., & Conaglen, J. V. (2003). Sexual desire in women presenting for antiandrogen therapy. *Journal of Sex & Marital Therapy, 29*, 255–267.

Cwikel, J., Gidron, Y., & Sheiner, E. (2004). Psychological interactions with infertility among women. *European Journal of Obstetrics & Gynecology and Reproductive Biology, 117*(2), 126–131.

D'Anna, R., Di Benedetto, V., Rizzo, P., Raffone, E., Interdonato, M. L., Corrado, F., & Di Benedetto, A. (2012). Myo-inositol may prevent gestational diabetes in PCOS women. *Gynecological Endocrinology, 28*(6), 440–442.

D'Anna, R., Scilipoti, A., Giordano, D., Caruso, C., Cannata, M. L., Interdonato, M. L., ... Di Benedetto, A. (2013). myo-Inositol supplementation and onset of gestational diabetes mellitus in pregnant women with a family history of type 2 diabetes: A prospective, randomized, placebo-controlled study. *Diabetes Care, 36*(4), 854–857.

de Niet, J. E., Pastoor, H., Timman, R., & Laven, J. S. E. (2012). Psycho-social and sexual well-being in women with polycystic ovary syndrome. In S. Mukherjee (Ed.), *Polycystic Ovary Syndrome.* Rotterdam: IntechOpen.

Deeks, A. A., Gibson-Helm, M. E., & Teede, H. J. (2010). Anxiety and depression in polycystic ovary syndrome: A comprehensive investigation. *Fertility and Sterility, 93*(7), 2421–2423.

Demyttenaere, K., Nijs, P., Evers-Kiebooms, G., & Koninckx, P. R. (1992). Coping and the ineffectiveness of coping influence the outcome of in vitro fertilization through stress responses. *Psychoneuroendocrinology, 17*, 655–665.

Dokras, A., Sarwer, D. B., Allison, K. C., Milman, L., Kris-Etherton, P. M., Kunselman, A. R., ... Fleming, J. (2016). Weight loss and lowering androgens predict improvements in health-related quality of life in women with PCOS. *The Journal of Clinical Endocrinology & Metabolism, 101*(8), 2966–2974.

Domar, A. D., Clapp, D., Slawsby, E., Kessel, B., Orav, J., & Freizinger, M. (2000). The impact of group psychological interventions on distress in infertile women. *Health Psychology, 19*(6), 568.

Ecklund, L. C., & Usadi, R. S. (2015). Endocrine and reproductive effects of poly-cystic ovarian syndrome. *Obstetrics and Gynecology Clinics of North America, 42*, 55–65.

Ercan, C. M., Coksuer, H., Aydogan, U., Alanbay, I., Keskin, U., Karasahin, K. E., & Baser, I. (2013). Sexual dysfunction assessment and hormonal correlations in patients with polycystic ovary syndrome. *International Journal of Impotence Research, 25*, 127–132.

Gold, S. M., Schulz, H., Mönch, A., Schulz, K. H., & Heesen, C. (2003). Cognitive impairment in multiple sclerosis does not affect reliability and validity of self-report health measures. *Multiple Sclerosis, 9*, 404–410.

Graham, A., & Hamoda, H. (2016). Treatment of polycystic ovarian syndrome in primary care. *Prescriber, 27*(11), 36–45.

Hadley, R. A., Newby, C., & Barry, J. A. (2019). Anxious childhood attachment predicts childlessness in later life. *Psychreg Journal of Psychology, 4*(2), 1–14.

Himelein, M. J., & Thatcher, S. S. (2006). Depression and body image among women with polycystic ovary syndrome. *Journal of Health Psychology, 11*, 613–625.

Hosaka, T., Matsubayashi, H., Sugiyama, Y., Izumi, S. I., & Makino, T. (2002). Effect of psychiatric group intervention on natural-killer cell activity and pregnancy rate. *General Hospital Psychiatry, 24*(5), 353–356.

Jacobs, M. B., Boynton-Jarrett, R. D., & Harville, E. W. (2015). Adverse childhood event experiences, fertility difficulties and menstrual cycle characteristics. *Journal of Psychosomatic Obstetrics and Gynecology, 36*(2), 46–57.

Jayasena, C. N., & Franks, S. (2014). The management of patients with polycystic ovary syndrome. *Nature Reviews Endocrinology, 10*(10), 624.

Kitzinger, C., & Willmott, J. (2002). 'The thief of womanhood': Women's experience of polycystic ovarian syndrome. *Social Science & Medicine, 54*, 349–361.

Klonoff-Cohen, H., Chu, E., Natarajan, L., & Sieber, W. (2001). A prospective study of stress among women undergoing in vitro fertilization or gamete intrafallopian transfer. *Fertility and Sterility, 76,* 675–687.

Levitas, E., Parmet, A., Lunenfeld, E., Bentov, Y., Burstein, E., Friger, M., & Potashnik, G. (2006). Impact of hypnosis during embryo transfer on the outcome of in vitro fertilization–embryo transfer: a case-control study. *Fertility and Sterility, 85*(5), 1404–1408.

Løvvik, T. S., Carlsen, S. M., Salvesen, Ø., Steffensen, B., Bixo, M., Gómez-Real, F., … Trouva, A. (2019). Use of metformin to treat pregnant women with polycystic ovary syndrome (PregMet2): A randomised, double-blind, placebo-controlled trial. *The Lancet Diabetes & Endocrinology, 7*(4), 256–266.

Mącik, D. (2016). Loss of attributes of femininity, anxiety and value crisis. Women with polycystic ovary syndrome compared to women after mastectomy and in menopause. *Health Psychology Report, 4*(2), 159–169.

March, W. A., Whitrow, M. J., Davies, M. J., Fernandez, R. C., & Moore, V. M. (2018). Postnatal depression in a community-based study of women with polycystic ovary syndrome. *Acta Obstetricia et Gynecologica Scandinavica, 97*(7), 838–844.

Matsubayashi, H., Shida, M., Kondo, A., Suzuki, T., Sugi, T., Izumi, S. I., … Makino, T. (2005). Preconception peripheral natural killer cell activity as a predictor of pregnancy outcome in patients with unexplained infertility. *American Journal of Reproductive Immunology, 53*(3), 126–131.

McCook, J. G. (2002). *The influence of hyperandrogenism, obesity and infertility on the psychosocial health and wellbeing of women with polycystic ovary syndrome.* Unpublished doctoral dissertation, University of Michigan.

McCook, J. G., Reame, N. E., & Thatcher, S. S. (2005). Health-related quality of life issues in women with polycystic ovary syndrome. *Journal of Obstetric, Gynecologic, and Neonatal Nursing, 34,* 12–20.

Milazzo, A., Mnatzaganian, G., Elshaug, A. G., Hemphill, S. A., Hiller, J. E., & Astute Health Study Group. (2016). Depression and anxiety outcomes associated with failed assisted reproductive technologies: A systematic review and meta-analysis. *PLoS One, 11*(11), e0165805.

Morotti, E., Persico, N., Battaglia, B., Fabbri, R., Meriggiola, M. C., Venturoli, S., & Battaglia, C. (2013). Body imaging and sexual behavior in lean women with polycystic ovary syndrome. *The Journal of Sexual Medicine, 10*(11), 2752–2760.

Murgel, A. C. F., Simões, R. S., Maciel, G. A. R., Soares, J. M., Jr., & Baracat, E. C. (2019). Sexual dysfunction in women with polycystic ovary syndrome: Systematic review and meta-analysis. *The Journal of Sexual Medicine, 16*(4), 542–550.

NICE. (2019a). *Clomifene citrate.* BNF. Retrieved May 5, 2019, from https://bnf.nice.org.uk/drug/clomifene-citrate.html.

NICE. (2019b). *Co-cyprindiol.* Retrieved May 12, 2019, from https://bnf.nice.org.uk/drug/co-cyprindiol.html.

Owen, R., & Jobling, S. (2012). Environmental science: The hidden costs of flexible fertility. *Nature, 485*(7399), 441.

Pastoor, H., Timman, R., de Klerk, C., Bramer, W. M., Laan, E. T., & Laven, J. S. (2018). Sexual function in women with polycystic ovary syndrome: A systematic review and meta-analysis. *Reproductive Biomedicine Online, 37*(6), 750–760.

Qu, F., Wu, Y., Zhu, Y. H., Barry, J., Ding, T., Baio, G., … Hardiman, P. J. (2017). The association between psychological stress and miscarriage: A systematic review and meta-analysis. *Scientific Reports, 7*(1), 1731.

Rellini, A. H., Stratton, N., Tonani, S., Santamaria, V., Brambilla, E., & Nappi, R. E. (2013). Differences in sexual desire between women with clinical versus biochemical signs of hyperandrogenism in polycystic ovarian syndrome. *Hormones and Behavior, 63*(1), 65–71.

Rivest, S., & Rivier, C. (1995). The role of corticotropin-releasing factor and interleukin-1 in the regulation of neurons controlling reproductive functions. *Endocrine Reviews, 16*, 177–199.

Robinson, S. A., Dowell, M., Pedulla, D., & McCauley, L. (2004). Do the emotional side-effects of hormonal contraceptives come from pharmacologic or psychological mechanisms? *Medical Hypotheses, 63*(2), 268–273.

Sarrel, P. M., & DeCherney, A. H. (1985). Psychotherapeutic intervention for treatment of couples with secondary infertility. *Fertility and Sterility, 43*, 897–900.

Selye, H. (1950). Stress and the general adaptation syndrome. *British medical journal, 1*(4667), 1383.

Smeenk, J. M. J., Verhaak, C. M., Eugster, A., Van Minnen, A., Zielhuis, G. A., & Braat, D. D. M. (2001). The effect of anxiety and depression on the outcome of in-vitro fertilization. *Human Reproduction, 16*(7), 1420–1423.

Smeenk, J. M. J., Verhaak, C. M., Vingerhoets, A. J. J. M., Sweep, C. G. J., Merkus, J. M. W. M., Willemsen, S. J., … Braat, D. D. M. (2005). Stress and outcome success in IVF: The role of self-reports and endocrine variables. *Human Reproduction, 20*(4), 991–996.

Stapinska-Syniec, A., Grabowska, K., Szpotanska-Sikorska, M., & Pietrzak, B. (2018). Depression, sexual satisfaction, and other psychological issues in women with polycystic ovary syndrome. *Gynecological Endocrinology, 34*(7), 597–600.

Stovall, D. W., Scriver, J. L., Clayton, A. H., Williams, C. D., & Pastore, L. M. (2012). Sexual function in women with polycystic ovary syndrome. *The Journal of Sexual Medicine, 9*(1), 224–230.

Sullivan, M. (2017, August 31). What's in a name? *Clinical Endocrinology News.*

Sullivan, E. A., Zegers-Hochschild, F., Mansour, R., Ishihara, O., De Mouzon, J., Nygren, K. G., & Adamson, G. D. (2013). International Committee for Monitoring Assisted Reproductive Technologies (ICMART) world report: Assisted reproductive technology 2004. *Human Reproduction, 28*(5), 1375–1390.

Tan, S., Hahn, S., Benson, S., Janssen, O. E., Dietz, T., Kimmig, R., … Elsenbruch, S. (2008). Psychological implications of infertility in women with polycystic ovary syndrome. *Human Reproduction, 23*(9), 2064–2071.

Tang, T., Lord, J. M., Norman, R. J., Yasmin, E., & Balen, A. H. (2012). Insulin sensitising drugs (metformin, rosiglitazone, pioglitazone, D-chiro-inositol) for women with polycystic ovary syndrome, oligo amenorrhoea and subfertility. *The Cochrane Database of Systematic Reviews, 5*, CD003053. Retrieved from http://onlinelibrary.wiley.com/doi/10.1002/14651858.CD003053. pub5/abstract20.

Trent, M. E., Rich, M., Austin, S. B., & Gordon, C. M. (2003). Fertility concerns and sexual behavior in adolescent girls with polycystic ovary syndrome: Implications for quality of life. *Journal of Pediatric and Adolescent Gynecology, 16*(1), 33–37.

van Wely, M., Bayram, N., Bossuyt, P. M., & van der Veen, F. (2004). Laparoscopic electrocautery of the ovaries versus recombinant FSH in clomiphene citrate-resistant polycystic ovary syndrome. Impact on women's health-related quality of life. *Human Reproduction, 19*, 2244–2250.

Yu, Q., Hu, S., Wang, Y., Cheng, G., Xia, W., & Zhu, C. (2019). Letrozole versus laparoscopic ovarian drilling in clomiphene citrate-resistant women with polycystic ovary syndrome: A systematic review and meta-analysis of randomized controlled trials. *Reproductive Biology and Endocrinology, 17*(1), 17.

Zueff, L. N., Lara, L. A. D. S., Vieira, C. S., Martins, W. D. P., & Ferriani, R. A. (2015). Body composition characteristics predict sexual functioning in obese women with or without PCOS. *Journal of Sex & Marital Therapy, 41*(3), 227–237.

7

Psychobiological Pathways of PCOS

Abstract From the preceding chapters of this book, readers will by now know that the psychology of PCOS is seldom straightforward. In this chapter you will see how the various strands of evidence can be pulled together in a way that makes sense of the overall psychobiological picture of PCOS—from prenatal development, and throughout the lifespan. Several pathways are described, and the evidence for four pathways is explored, including the evidence for how a person's mental state can impact biology, and why this can be so important in PCOS.

Keywords Organisational effect • Activational effect • Mechanism • Prenatal • Lifespan

Introduction

It is recognised that our knowledge of the biological underpinnings of the psychological issues related to PCOS is in its infancy (Papalou and Diamanti-Kandarakis 2017). There is more than one mechanism of action at work, and the multiplicity of pathways is complex. There is probably a

© The Author(s) 2019

J. A. Barry, *Psychological Aspects of Polycystic Ovary Syndrome*,

https://doi.org/10.1007/978-3-030-30290-0_7

tendency to be less inclined to precisely identify a mechanism of action when the results are impressive and reliable, the mechanisms in PCOS are not so clear. Nonetheless, understanding the mechanisms and pathways involved has important implications for our understanding of PCOS, and our ability to treat this condition more effectively.

An example of the complexity of the action of testosterone on the fetus is demonstrated by the relatively recent finding that AMH is probably the key variable in the prenatal androgenisation of the fetus (Tata et al. 2018). Although it has been long suspected that prenatal androgenisation is at the root of PCOS (Abbott et al. 2002; Barry et al. 2010), the precise pathway had remained somewhat elusive (see below, or Chap. 1 for a description of the AMH mechanism).

The uncertainties and complexities of PCOS require that scientists generate testable hypotheses. In response to this need, the material presented in this chapter is more theoretical and speculative than the other chapters. The model proposed by Barry et al. (2018) in the journal *Medical Hypotheses*, based on Barry (2011), is—I hope—a useful step forward. This biopsychological model (described below in Figs. 7.1, 7.2, and 7.3) suggests ways to interpret the phenomena that we see in PCOS. The complexity of the pathways is underlined by the fact that causality goes not only from biology to psychology, but from psychology to biology.

This first part of this chapter will explore four psychobiological pathways, describe evidence for them, and suggest how understanding the underlying mechanisms can help us to develop effective treatment strategies. The second part of this chapter will focus more closely on perhaps the most important pathway: how prenatal androgenisation might occur in PCOS.

Four Ways That Testosterone Makes an Impact

Testosterone has an impact on biology and psychology in different ways.

- *Organisational effects* occur prenatally and cause permanent changes to biological structures. In humans and other mammals, neurobehavioural sexual differentiation occurs early in development and involves permanent changes in neural structures and behaviour (Hines 2009).

- *Activational effects* are ephemeral and are caused by testosterone in the bloodstream. They may cause changes to neural structures, though less permanent than organisational effects, and can be reversed by cessation of exposure to hormones. For example, testosterone has a strong activational effect on gene expression in mouse stem cells, but this effect ceases when exposure to testosterone ceases (Bramble et al. 2016).
- *Direct effects* occur when testosterone acts directly upon receptors or other aspects of biology without mediation or moderation of other factors. In practice, it can be difficult to identify direct effects with certainty because of the complexity of the endocrine and other systems.
- *Indirect effects* occur where the impact of testosterone is mediated by another variable. For example, sometimes the masculinising effect of testosterone on neural development only occurs after testosterone has been converted to estadiol (Roselli 2007). Several examples from PCOS research are given below, where the effect of testosterone on distress is mediated by how much testosterone has an impact on aspects of PCOS, such as obesity, which cause distress.

These effects may be complex; for example, an effect can be both direct and activational. Because of this complexity it can be difficult to say if a pathway is truly direct, or whether it just appears to be direct because we have not identified other elements that are involved. This can occur even with very strong correlations that appear to show a causal relationship, when in fact, the relationship is fully mediated by a third variable.

In this chapter, evidence is presented that testosterone impacts women with PCOS in various ways: (1) mental rotation ability is enhanced via a direct and activational pathway to neuroreceptors; (2) when distress is caused by the physiological symptoms of testosterone (e.g. acne), this is via an indirect and activational pathway; (3) when low mood in PCOS is caused by low blood sugar, this is via an indirect and organisational effect. (4) Perhaps most interesting of all, the direction of causality can be reversed, such as the case when deep relaxation can cause a reduction in adrenal androgens (substances with a testosterone-like effect).

The model described in below Figs. 7.1, 7.2, and 7.3 is based on findings from research from a variety of sources, mainly PCOS, congenital adrenal hyperplasia (CAH), and animal research. The model was originally described by Barry (2011), and Barry et al. (2018).

Visuo-spatial Ability in PCOS Is Enhanced by Testosterone: A Direct and Activational Effect

The three-dimensional mental rotation task is a puzzle-like test in which participants are asked to look at a drawing ('figure') of a stack of cubes, then compare these to four other similar-looking stacks of cubes. The task is to identify which of the four figures is the same as the first figure. Two of the figures are the same as the first, but are seen from a different angle (i.e. 'rotated'), and the other two figures are not the same as the first. The difficulty is that to do this you need to imagine what the various figures would look like if viewed from different angles. If the figures were to come to life and you could hold them in your hand, rotating each in turn and seeing them from various angles, the task would be much simpler, but participants in this test are being asked to make comparisons using only their imagination: hence, 'mental rotation'.

In general, men perform significantly better on this task than women do (Peters et al. 1995). This seems to be related to men having greater levels of testosterone than women (usually about 10 times more), and in support of this, it has been found that a single dose of testosterone can improve scoring on this task in women (Aleman et al. 2004), demonstrating a direct activational effect of testosterone.

Because women with PCOS often have higher levels of testosterone than other women, you would probably predict that women with PCOS are better at mental rotation than other women. Barry et al. (2013) tested this hypothesis in a study of 69 women with PCOS and 41 subfertile control women. All participants completed the standard Shepard-Metzler three-dimensional mental rotation task (Shepard and Metzler 1971). It was found that the median scores of women with PCOS (median = 3.00) were higher than controls (median = 2.00) ($p < 0.047$). In the PCOS group but not controls, testosterone was positively correlated with mental rotation scores ($r_s = 0.376$, $p < 0.002$), and estradiol (the main estrogen) was negatively correlated with mental rotation scores ($r_s = -0.473$, $p < 0.010$). Other factors, including general intelligence and social class, did not explain these results. These findings suggest that mental rotation ability was the result of a direct activational effect of testosterone in women with PCOS (Fig. 7.1).

It could be suggested that organisational effects also have a role to play, because it is possible that prenatal exposure to testosterone in PCOS pregnancies (Barry et al. 2010) masculinises brain morphology (Fig. 7.1). According to this hypothesis, prenatal exposure increases the expression of androgen receptors in regions associated with visuo-spatial ability (cortical areas, the hippocampus, and parietal lobe). The increased number of receptors would facilitate the uptake of circulating testosterone, increasing mental rotation task performance. Counter to the organisational

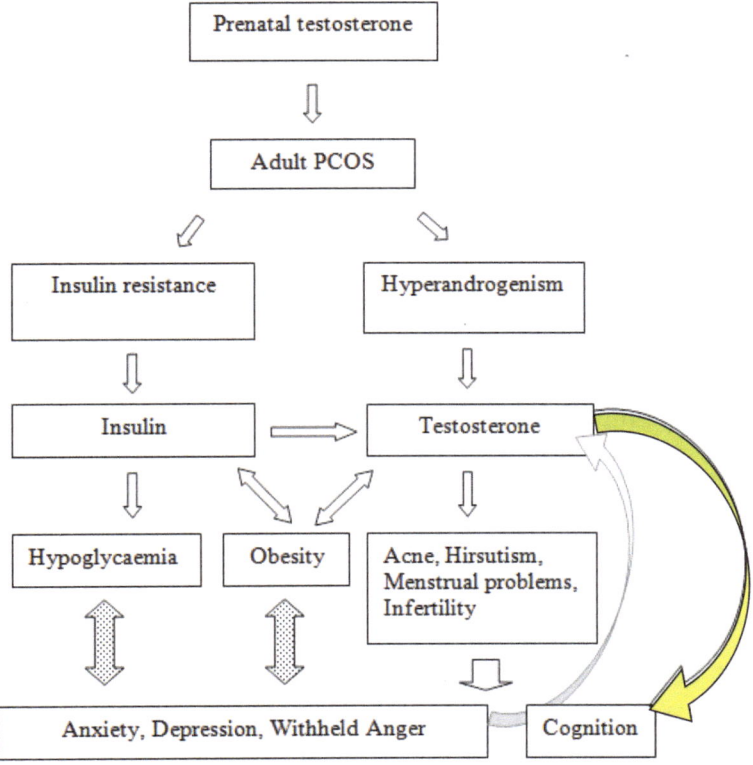

Fig. 7.1 A model of the suggested pathway (highlighted in yellow) underlying mental rotation ability in PCOS. Note that this direct and activational pathway may stem from the prenatal organisation of brain development in areas associated with mental rotation ability (not shown in diagram), which would be an indirect/organisational effect

explanation, however, is the fact that Barry et al. (2013) found that only the women with PCOS who had higher levels of circulating testosterone showed enhanced mental rotation ability. Further research (as suggested by Barry et al. 2013) would be useful in addressing the question of pre-natal exposure to testosterone, which has important implications for our understanding of the role of prenatal androgens in PCOS development.

Another interesting aspect of the mental rotation and testosterone in PCOS is that there is evidence that testosterone is a double-edged sword, in that although it might help with mental rotation ability, the additional impact of testosterone on anxiety in PCOS might work against the ability to perform well under test conditions (see section on *Testosterone and cognition* in Chap. 4).

This phenomenon is also interesting in terms of another type of pathway; fMRI scans have shown the activation of different *neural* pathways in men and women (see overview by Barry and Owens 2019). Men tend to show activation in the parietal areas, whereas women show activation in the right inferior frontal area. The difference in neural pathway activation might be caused by men and women using different solving strategies, with men using a coordinate processing approach and women using a serial categorical processing approach. These differ-ent neural pathways and approaches might be the result of prenatal androgenisation of the brain typically experienced by the male fetus, perhaps creating more androgen receptors in the parietal areas than occurs in female fetal development.

Some of the Anxiety and Depression Seen in PCOS May Be Caused by Testosterone, But Only When Symptoms Caused by Testosterone Are Experienced as Unpleasant: An Indirect Activational Effect of Testosterone

It seems intuitively correct that because testosterone causes the PCOS symptoms that women find distressing, higher testosterone levels will lead to distress. For example, we know that obesity generally has an impact on anxiety and depression in PCOS; Barry et al. (2011) found that anxiety and depression were slightly worse in women with a higher BMI (a Hedge's g difference of around 0.14). However, there are individual differences in sensitivity to androgen (Vottero et al. 1999). The implications of this are that some women can have relatively high levels of testosterone without it having much impact on their PCOS symptoms. Furthermore, people vary in how much they are bothered by PCOS symptoms. For example, Hashimoto et al. (2003) found that Austrian women with PCOS are more concerned about obesity issues than hirsutism issues. For these reasons—and perhaps also others, such as the accuracy of some testosterone assays—there is not a very consistent correlation between testosterone and symptoms of PCOS (Legro et al. 2010), nor testosterone and QoL for symptoms of PCOS (Barry et al. 2018). This isn't to say that there is no relationship between testosterone and distress in PCOS; just that the relationship is complicated. So, what is the pathway between testosterone and distress in PCOS?

A study by Barry et al. (2011b) assessed the degree to which testosterone is implicated in mood in PCOS. Seventy-six women with PCOS and 49 subfertile control women completed the HADS, PCOSQ, EPQ, and the STAXI. There was little evidence of a correlation (either linear or nonlinear) between testosterone and mood. Similarly, Enjezab et al. (2017) found no correlation between testosterone and depression in women with PCOS—in fact, the correlation was weakly negative ($r = -0.16$; $n = 62$; $p < 0.31$). Most well-designed studies have also found no significant correlation between testosterone and depression in PCOS (e.g. Rahiminejad et al. 2014). Two studies (Annagür et al. 2013; Klimczak et al. 2015) have reported an impact of adrenal androgens (but not testosterone) on depression, but because adrenal androgens are responsive to distress, it seems likely that the depression caused the elevation in adrenal androgens, and not visa-versa. (See also the final pathway described below, from body to mind.)

A re-analysis by Barry et al. (2018) of the data by Barry et al. (2011b) showed that although testosterone was weakly correlated with mood, how badly women felt about their PCOS symptoms was much more strongly correlated with mood. Similarly, Greenwood et al. (2018) found that depressed women with PCOS reported worse QoL for mood, weight, menstrual problems, infertility, and body hair.

Bearing in mind that PCOS symptoms are caused by testosterone, these findings suggest that mood in PCOS is influenced by an indirect activational effect of testosterone. In other words, testosterone causes the physical symptoms associated with PCOS (acne, menstrual problems etc.), but it is *the degree to which these symptoms are perceived as unpleasant* that will dictate the degree to which the symptoms impact mood (Fig. 7.2, yellow pathway).

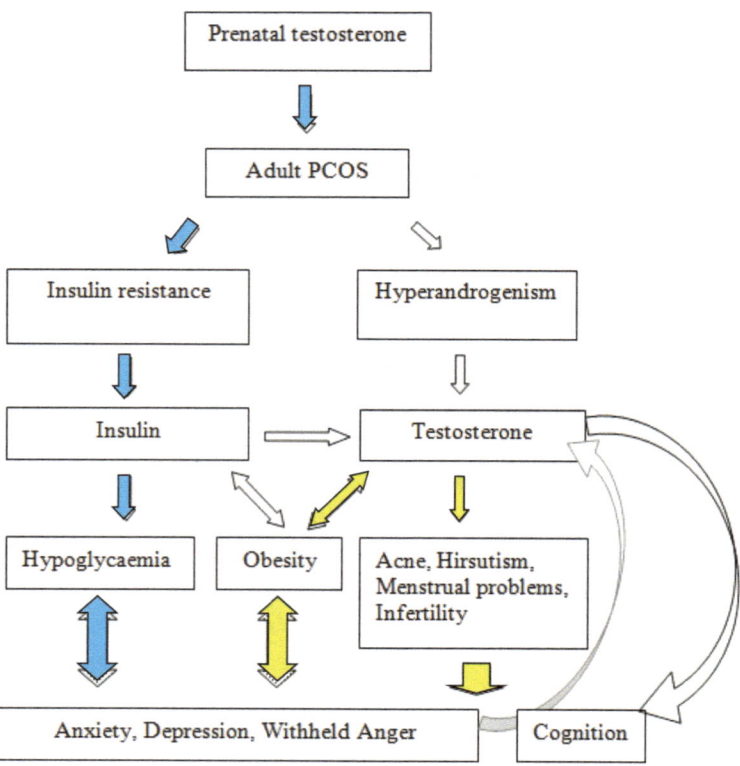

Fig. 7.2 Model of the suggested pathways underlying mood problems in PCOS. Mood problems might be caused indirectly by testosterone via increasing the distressing symptoms of PCOS (highlighted in yellow). Mood problems might also be caused by the prenatal organisation of the metabolism, resulting in reactive hypoglycaemia, an indirect/organisational effect of testosterone and a direct/activational effect of low blood glucose (highlighted in blue)

A similar pathway was described in a study of the correlation between testosterone and anger in male-to-female transsexuals and female-to-male transsexuals (Defreyne et al. 2019; see Chap. 4).

Anxiety and Depression in PCOS Can Be Caused by Low Blood Sugar, Which In Turn Is The Result of Prenatal Testosterone: An Organisational Effect

Glucose is used by the brain for energy, and the brain needs about 125–150 grams per day to function properly. Most of the glucose the brain and body use comes from food. If blood sugars become critically low (a state called *hypoglycaemia*), this can result in a state called 'tense-tiredness' in which the person feels anxious, depressed, and tired (Thayer 1989). Experimental induction of hypoglycaemia in healthy participants reliably causes this tense-tired mood state (e.g. Gold et al. 1995).

Why is this relevant to PCOS? Well, firstly we know that women with PCOS are more likely to experience anxiety and depression—which are two of the three symptoms of tense-tiredness—than other women. The third symptom of tense-tiredness—fatigue—is, according to Hollinrake et al. (2007), one of the most commonly reported symptoms of depression in women with PCOS. Unfortunately it is not often asked about specifically in research. Secondly, there is evidence that women with PCOS show more of the psychological signs associated with hypoglycaemia than other women do (Barry et al. 2011a), including signs of tense-tiredness. In fact women with PCOS are at least 4 times more likely than other women to experience 'reactive hypoglycaemia', a state of lowered blood glucose experienced after meals (Altuntas et al. 2005; Kasim-Karakas et al. 2007).

Reactive hypoglycaemia is quite an interesting phenomenon, especially for women with PCOS (see more detail in Chap. 5 of this book), not only because it might explain some of their low mood, but also because it suggests a solution based on a diet that moderates the amount of glucose in the bloodstream, known as the low-GI diet (see Chap. 5). Unfortunately, it is reported anecdotally that in some countries, such as the UK, physicians are sceptical that such symptoms are caused by hypoglycaemia, even though this can be diagnosed with a simple 5-hour oral glucose tolerance (OGTT) test.

But how does this relate to testosterone? Well, the answer demonstrates the complexity of the pathways in the relationship between testosterone and mood: it is possible that in PCOS pregnancies there is an organisational effect of elevated prenatal testosterone on the metabolic system of the developing fetus, resulting in insulin resistance and glucose imbalance in adulthood (Fig. 7.2, above—blue pathway). This pathway, for the time being at least, remains an untested hypothesis although it is supported by animal models which demonstrate a link between elevated prenatal testosterone and the development of a PCOS phenotype in later life (Abbott et al. 2002, 2019). In one way this phenomenon also demonstrates a direct effect of glucose, but in the context of the present chapter we are interested in the pathway related to testosterone.

Obesity is also a factor relevant to this discussion. Reactive hypoglycaemia (typically mid-afternoon) may contribute to weight gain in PCOS (Magnotti and Futterweit 2007); this could occur because insulin induces the production of androgens such as testosterone, which in turn increase visceral fat (Stanley and Misra 2008). Reactive hypoglycaemia has been described as one of the 'subtle symptoms' of PCOS (Brand-Miller et al. 2004, p. 9) and a low glycemic index (GI) diet may be a way of controlling this problem. The relationship between hypoglycaemia, tense-tiredness, and obesity might explain the correlation between insulin resistance and depression sometimes seen in PCOS (Greenwood et al. 2015, 2018).

Learning to Relax Can Reduce Stress Hormones and Adrenal Androgens

It has become common knowledge that when people become distressed, they release stress hormones, such as adrenaline and cortisol, from the adrenal glands. A-level psychology students are taught about the psychobiological pathway from the hypothalamus to the adrenal glands via adrenocorticotropic hormone (ACTH), and many people are familiar with the term 'fight or flight' response.

However some lesser known facts are relevant. Firstly, women with PCOS are more inclined to experience anxiety than are other women. Secondly, when activated, the adrenal glands produce not only stress hormones like adrenalin and cortisol, but adrenal androgens—testosterone-like substances. Furthermore, women with PCOS may be more sensitive to ACTH, potentially leading to an even higher level of production of adrenal androgens than women experiencing similar levels of distress (McKenna and Cunningham 1995; Milutinović et al. 2011; Moran et al. 2004). Taking this information together, the conclusion is that a vicious cycle may occur, whereby the distress that women with PCOS experience may be contributing to their androgen levels, thus increasing their distressing symptoms.

However there exists a positive side to this. The fight or flight response has its corollary—the 'relaxation response'. This is the inverse of the fight or flight response, where the physiological responses slow down and reduce their activity, including a reduction in adrenal gland activity, and reduction of substances thereof. In other words, when someone starts to relax, adrenal androgen production starts to reduce.

This obviously has positive implications for women with PCOS, in that a reduction in distress might lead to a reduction in the overall burden of androgens in PCOS. This mechanism has been tested in a pilot study of 13 women with PCOS (Barry et al. 2017). In this study, it was found that inducing relaxation using a talking-based treatment (progressive muscle relaxation and guided imagery) not only reduced levels of adrenal androgens, but also reduced anxiety and depression levels. This study (described in more detail in Chap. 8) demonstrates that the causal pathway from body to mind can work the other way too—from mind to body—via a direct activational effect (see Fig. 7.3).

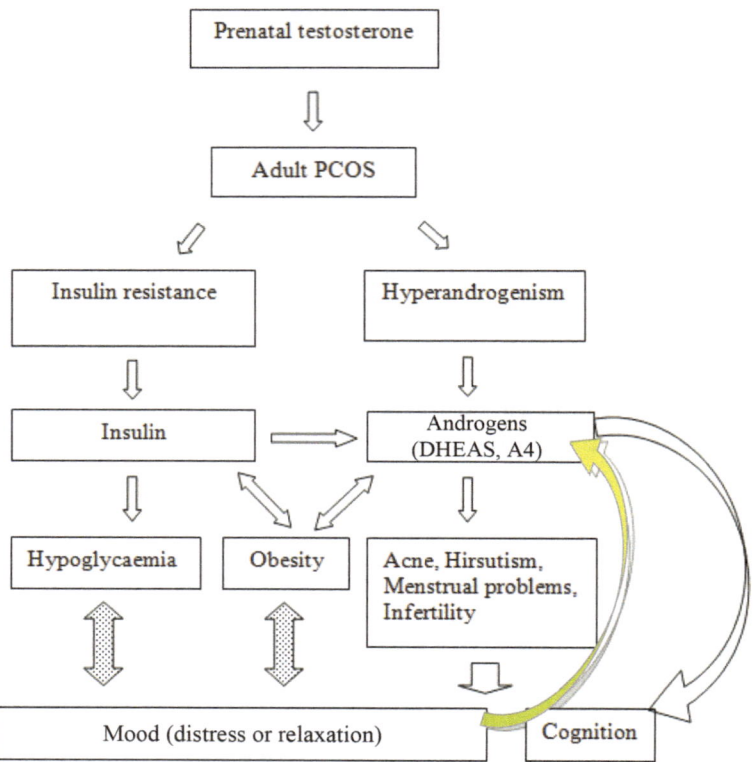

Fig. 7.3 A model of the suggested pathway (highlighted in yellow) underlying the reduction of adrenal androgens in PCOS. This is likely to be a direct activational effect of psychological relaxation reducing the activity of the adrenal glands (not shown in diagram), thus reducing the production of adrenal androgens (DHEAS and androstenedione) as well as the adrenal hormone cortisol

An Exploration of How Prenatal Testosterone Might Cause PCOS

Perhaps the most important pathway in PCOS is the one that leads to this syndrome in the first place. An excellent review of the literature on this topic concluded the 'evidence suggests that the intrauterine environment in pregnant PCOS women is hyperandrogenic' and that the most likely cause of the hyperandrogenism was a 'dysfunctional placenta', with AMH playing an 'enigmatic role in PCOS pathogenesis' (Filippou and Homburg 2017, p. 428). Subsequent evidence (Tata et al. 2018) appears to confirm that the main source of the dysfunction in the placenta is AMH.

AMH and Prenatal Androgenisation

Although in the past there has been some interesting speculation that the cause of PCOS was a defect in the fetal ovary (Franks et al. 2006), the most likely explanation currently available is that anti-Müllerian hormone (AMH) weakens the ability of the placenta to prevent testosterone from crossing over to the fetus (Tata et al. 2018). As described in Chap. 1, pregnant women with PCOS have higher maternal serum AMH than healthy women. Because AMH disrupts the bioconversion of androgens to estrogens, women with PCOS have higher testosterone levels during pregnancy. Normally the placenta would act as a barrier to maternal testosterone impacting the fetus, but AMH allows the fetus to be exposed to elevated testosterone levels because AMH inhibits the expression of aromatase in the placenta that converts testosterone to estradiol, the main estrogen, which is relatively harmless to female fetal development. Figure 7.4 illustrates how disruption of normal conversion of maternal testosterone to estradiol could lead to the fetus being exposed to elevated testosterone levels.

There are a few things to note about the mechanism illustrated here. Firstly, it is hypothetical: we do not know exactly how this process works, but Fig. 7.4 offers a simplified illustration a plausible scenario. Secondly, regardless of the mechanism, being exposed to elevated testosterone is far less problematic for the male fetus than the female fetus. That is because in healthy pregnancies (and probably in PCOS pregnancies too) typically the male fetal testicles release a huge surge of testosterone at around prenatal weeks 8–24 (Smail et al. 1981), exposing the male fetus to levels of testosterone similar to levels seen normally again at puberty in the male. Even at the end of pregnancy many weeks after the testosterone surge has

a

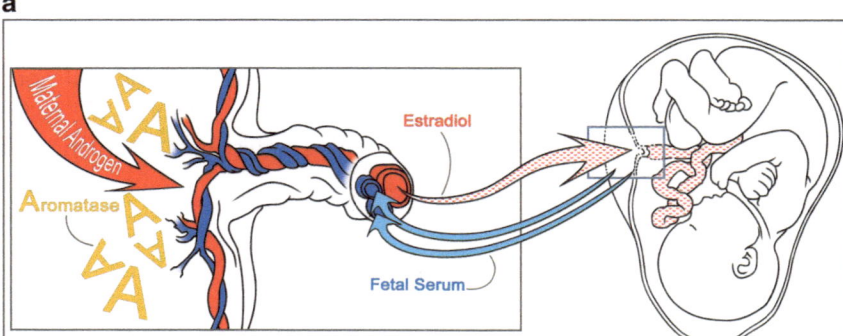

b

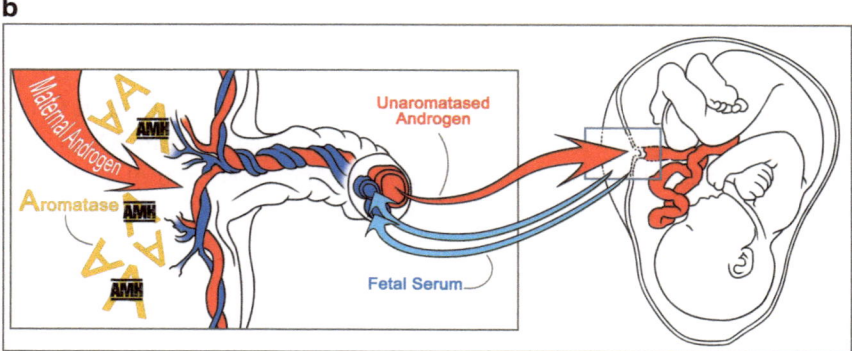

Fig. 7.4 Illustration of the hypothesised mechanism by which the female fetus in PCOS is exposed to elevated testosterone levels. The left side shows the placenta and umbilical cord, and the right side shows the fetus in the fetal sac connected by the umbilical cord to the placenta. The top section (**a**) shows a healthy pregnancy, where maternal testosterone is converted to estradiol by placental aromatase. The bottom section (**b**) shows what is hypothesised to happen in a PCOS pregnancy, where placental aromatase is impeded by AMH and therefore fails to convert some or all maternal testosterone to estradiol

ended, it is normal for testosterone levels to be higher in a male pregnancy compared to female, as shown by the levels of testosterone seen in the umbilical cord serum of healthy pregnancies (Barry et al. 2011). Thirdly, in the umbilical cord, there are two independent channels; blood in the arteries comes from the fetus, whereas blood in the vein comes from the placenta and may contain maternal products (Barry et al. 2011).

This third point is important with regard to research methodology for assessing the source of elevated testosterone in PCOS prenatally, because studies that take mixed samples (vein and arteries) from the umbilical cord will not be able to see how much testosterone is from the fetus and how much is of maternal/placental origin. Fourthly, note that unless stated otherwise, the research findings presented below are from healthy women (an indicator that more research focusing on PCOS is needed).

What is the evidence that a PCOS pregnancy is exposed to higher than normal levels of testosterone? One of the safest ways of testing whether the fetus in a PCOS pregnancy is exposed to elevated testosterone is to look at the levels of testosterone in the umbilical cord after the child has been delivered. Barry et al. (2010) found that testosterone levels in the umbilical cord of girls born to mothers with PCOS were surprisingly high—in fact, as high as those found in the umbilical cord of boys of healthy pregnancies. However, this study had a small sample size and used only a basic assay method, and although was replicated by a study using similar methodology (Maliqueo et al. 2013), studies using different methodologies have not replicated those findings. For example, a small study by Anderson et al. (2010) found no difference in cord blood between PCOS and healthy controls, but they used mixed cord blood samples, and the testosterone levels in 66% of their samples fell below the detection range of their assay. An interesting study (Carlsen and Vanky 2010) of the impact of metformin on pregnancy in PCOS didn't have a healthy control group, and presented data either by gender or by metformin status, so the crucial comparison could not be made of testosterone levels in girls with mothers with PCOS to girls of healthy mothers.

The Fetoplacental Unit

The placenta is the interface between the maternal and placental blood systems. Both blood systems are separate, but the barrier between them is extremely thin—particularly towards the end of pregnancy—and the exchange of substances like testosterone can occur by the classic membranous transport mechanisms, such as, for example, simple diffusion or osmosis (Embryology.ch 2007). Testosterone is much more likely to pass through placental structures than some other hormones implicated in PCOS (e.g. AMH) because: (a) testosterone has a relatively small molecular mass, and (b) testosterone, like estradiol, is highly lipid-soluble (Cefalu and Pardridge 2006); thus, can dissolve and permeate placental cellular membranes. However, when testosterone is bound to the protein SHBG (or albumin, another binding protein), this requires a more complex passage from serum to cell; thus, any maternal testosterone that reaches fetal circulation is likely to need to be free (unbound) testosterone (Bammann et al. 1980). Thus measures of free testosterone give a more accurate assessment of the amount that could cross the placenta, while measures of total testosterone (typically used in these studies) in the umbilical vein include unbound maternal testosterone that has escaped conversion to estradiol by the placenta. Therefore, although arterial testosterone is more likely to reflect mainly the contents of fetal circulation, umbilical vein testosterone will, to some degree, reflect the amount of maternal testosterone the fetus is exposed to.

Aromatase

Apart from the sex of the fetus, perhaps the factor that has the greatest potential impact on testosterone levels is the P450 enzyme aromatase. This is a cytochrome present in the placenta and other areas (gonads, brain, adipose tissue, liver, muscle, and hair). In normal circumstances only about 1% enzyme activity is necessary to prevent an impact on the fetus of maternal androgens (Holt 2005). Because of the efficiency of this conversion process we would expect testosterone levels in the umbilical cord vein to be quite low (Troisi et al. 2003). In laboratory conditions Zharikova et al. (2006) found that placental aromatase from healthy pregnancies converted testosterone to E2 at an increasing rate up to 400 nmol/L of testosterone, at which point, the conversion process evened out to a relatively steady rate of around 55 pmol/mg protein per minute.

However, the aromatisation process does not always work successfully. Conte et al. (1994) report a case of masculinisation of a female newborn due to the otherwise healthy mother having a molecular defect in her aromatase gene. Nestler (1987) found that insulin during pregnancy reduces the efficacy of aromatase in the placenta, which has obvious relevance to PCOS pregnancies. Previous evidence found either no evidence of CYP19 mutations in PCOS (Soderlund et al. 2005) or mixed evidence (Xita et al. 2008). Abbott et al. (2002) suggest that 'it is difficult to imagine that hyperandrogenism is commonly passed across the placenta from a mother with PCOS to a previously unaffected daughter' unless there was disruption of placental aromatisation of maternal testosterone, maternal stress, or malnutrition (Abbott et al. 2002, p. 2). However we can now state with more certainty that the problem is primarily with AMH, and not a defect in aromatase per se or other factors (Tata et al. 2018).

Other Factors That Influence Umbilical Cord Testosterone

The other factors that can potentially influence testosterone levels in the umbilical cord are of interest in discussions of PCOS. First of all, they may still potentially add to the issues created by AMH. Secondly, they should be accounted for in PCOS research so that they are not potentially confounding variables. As can be seen in the studies here, there are a variety of assay methods and units of measurement for testosterone (described in Chap. 4). I have included the testosterone levels as reported in the original papers, which, although don't compare between studies, at least give a sense of comparison within each study.

Many women with PCOS suffer from insulin resistance, and this can be exacerbated in pregnancy, becoming gestational diabetes. Nestler (1987) found that insulin during pregnancy reduces the efficacy of placental aromatase. Thus it seems that gestational diabetes is another factor that could potentially expose the fetus to maternal testosterone.

The numerical order of all live births and fetal deaths has been shown to affect testosterone levels; Maccoby et al. (1979) found that firstborn males had higher umbilical cord testosterone levels than their later siblings, especially if the next sibling was born soon after the first. The difference could not be attributed to duration of labour, birth weight, or maternal age.

Maternal stress is another potential influence on cord and maternal testosterone levels. The adrenal glands are activated by psychological distress, as some researchers (Reiche et al. 2004; Furuhashi et al. 1981) found higher cortisol in the cord serum of boys, which they attributed to the stress of labour and delivery. Adrenal activation stimulates not only cortisol, but the secretion of the DHEAS, which is a precursor of testosterone (Leowattana 2004). Thus any pregnancy complication that increases stress has the potential to increase androgen levels. For example, Bolton et al. (1989) found that for preterm girls born between weeks 33 and 37, umbilical vein testosterone (UVT) was higher than term births (mean 3.8 vs 2.8 nmol/L), though the small sample size (14 cases for this comparison) makes conclusions difficult to draw. Barry et al. (2010) found no significant effect of type of delivery or duration of labour on testosterone levels in the mothers (PCOS and healthy women) or UVT.

There are often weaknesses in studies in this topic. However, the small sample sizes seen in many studies are probably a consequence, in many cases, of the logistical difficulties of collecting umbilical cord samples because the time of birth—unless a planned caesarean section—can be difficult to predict and might be in the early hours of the morning when researchers are not on duty to collect cord samples. Another non-infrequent issue is a lack of control of relevant variables. For example, Demisch et al. (1968) didn't control for parity or how close to delivery samples were taken, and Mathur et al. (1980) did not present testosterone values separately for boys and girls. Nonetheless, the available evidence does not indicate that pregnancy complications reliably increase testosterone

Other factors might influence cord testosterone levels, but these are less easy to control. For example, the kisspeptin peptide has been shown to androgenise the fetus in animal studies (Filippou and Homburg 2017).

Animal Studies of Testosterone in Pregnancy

Although there can be problems with generalising from animal studies to humans, there is good research evidence that—in animals at least—the AMH issues discovered in PCOS are not a necessary condition for the creation of PCOS. Dumesic et al. (2007) review research in this area, and concluded that adult dysfunctional ovarian morphology can be programmed simply by prenatal exposure to testosterone. There are many animal studies that confirm this, for example, in rhesus monkeys (Abbott et al. 1998), sheep (Clarke et al. 1977; Birch et al. 2003; Manikkam et al. 2006), rats (Foecking et al. 2005), and mice (Sullivan and Moenter 2004). Resko and Ellinwood (1984) and Resko et al. (1987) induced polycystic ovaries and anovulation in the female offspring of rhesus monkey mothers given doses of testosterone that exposed the female fetus to testosterone at levels normally experienced by a male fetus. Rhesus mothers were injected with 10–15 mg of testosterone for 15–35 days. Rhesus gestation lasts for 165 days, and testosterone injections started either early (days 40–60) or late (100–115) in pregnancy. Regardless of whether they were exposed to testosterone early or late in gestation, the female offspring had double the risk of developing a PCOS-like phenotype (anovulation + polycystic ovaries). The risk of developing either symptom alone was tenfold for anovulation and double the risk of polycystic ovaries.

It is possible that although this direct transfer from maternal circulation to fetus exists in animals, it does not in humans due to possibly greater efficiency of the human aromatisation process. This possibility has not been tested experimentally, but some evidence (e.g. the case studies by Foulk et al. 1997; Bertalan et al. 2007) suggests that in healthy humans, the placenta provides an effective barrier in healthy pregnancies.

There are, for good reasons, ethical restrictions on experimentation in humans, so the research on primates (e.g. Resko and Ellinwood 1984; Resko et al. 1987) offers probably the best comparison to PCOS in humans available. The animal studies could perhaps be criticised for lacking ecological validity in that they expose female fetuses to testosterone levels that would be normally seen only in males. However, Beck-Peccoz et al. (1991) found in humans during the second trimester that 40% of female fetuses experience testosterone levels equivalent to those seen in the fetal male range for this gestational period; thus, the animal models might be, at least, comparable to this 40%. Whether these normally-occurring elevations are high enough to affect developmental programming in humans is unknown.

Birth Weight

Animal studies have found that birth weight is linked to prenatal androgenisation: Manikkam et al. (2006) found that giving 32 pregnant sheep doses of testosterone during the mid-pregnancy period reduced birth weight and increased postnatal catch-up growth compared to 16 no-treatment controls. Low birth weight is a marker of intrauterine grow retardation, and human infants being born <2500 grams is linked with the risk of developing a range of conditions in adulthood, including menstrual irregularities (de Zegher and Ibáñez 2006) and PCOS (Cresswell et al. 1997). In a retrospective study, Benítez et al. (2001) found that low birth weight was more prevalent in newborns of PCOS mothers than found in women with normal menstruation cycles. Although Sir-Petermann et al. (2005) did not replicate this, they found that newborns of mothers with PCOS were significantly smaller for gestational age than controls (defined as being below the 5th percentile) and the newborns that were large for gestational age (above the 90th percentile) in the PCOS group had a greater birth length—that is, the newborn was longer (although whether this was measured from crown-to-heel or crown-to-rump is not stated). The link between low birth weight and risk of later disease is especially strong when low birth weight is followed by what is called 'postnatal catch-up'—where newborns that are underweight experience a surge in growth postnatally, leading to childhood obesity (Ong et al. 2000).

Critical Periods of Exposure and Sampling Methods

The timing of the prenatal exposure to testosterone is also potentially important, though this topic is under-researched. The first trimester is crucial in fetal development, as this is the time when the fetal gonads are differentiated. Grumbach and Ducharme (1960) suggest that after the first trimester androgen exposure carries much lower risks to the female fetus due to its pattern of androgen receptor expression, which makes urogenital development no longer responsive to testosterone. Thus the first trimester would seem to be the time of most risk for the female fetus of overt virilisation. However Foulk et al. (1997) report a testosterone level of 11.1 nmol/L at 10.5 weeks of pregnancy; this testosterone level is unusually high, but there was no evidence of virilisation in the female newborn. Similarly, Bertalan et al.'s (2007) patient had a maternal testosterone level of 15.2 nmol/L at week 11, with no apparent effect on the female newborn.

It is possible that testosterone levels in the third trimester, and even the postnatal period, are important to cognitive development (Hines 2004), therefore the umbilical cord levels at birth could be of most relevance to later cognitive functioning—for example, ability on the three-dimensional mental rotation task (described above and in Chap. 4). Note however that the umbilical cord levels at birth cannot be interpreted as indicating the levels at any other stage of pregnancy.

Critical periods are difficult to research. In theory, samples could be taken from the umbilical cord at any point during gestation, though this carries risks for the fetus. An alternative to cord samples is taking a sample from amniotic fluid, the protective liquid, consisting of nutrients and fetal urine, which surrounds the fetus during pregnancy. Although amniotic fluid is the standard way to investigate the effects of early fetal androgen exposure, sampling carries risks to the fetus. There are other issues, for example, amniotic testosterone levels are influenced by the functioning of the fetal kidneys (van de Beek et al. 2004). Also, testosterone levels from amniotic fluid are not comparable to those found in cord testosterone at the end of gestation because amniotic testosterone is usually sampled around weeks 11–21, when a sex difference in testosterone is likely to be the largest because of the testosterone surge in male fetuses (Smail et al. 1981). Furthermore, samples from amniotic fluid are usually taken because there are specific concerns about fetal development, so may also not be comparable to samples taken from the umbilical cord in the general population. Research into the impact of testosterone and other substances prenatally would be vastly improved if there were a safe way to take samples across the gestational period.

Why Is Learning About the Pathways Useful?

Having a greater understanding of the mechanism, or pathway of action, has several benefits. Firstly and most obviously, clinical interventions might be developed and tested. Secondly, identifying mechanisms leads to hypothesis development so that the validity of the mechanisms can be tested. Each new mechanism identified is a step further in understanding the pathway. Each new level of understanding is a platform from which further understanding, and clinical applications, can be developed. Thirdly, research in PCOS is most likely to work best when interdisciplinary teams of gynaecologists, psychologists, endocrinologists, and others collaborate in an open and a creative fashion. It is likely that the synergy of such combinations will create unexpected spin-off activities and discoveries.

Conclusions

For those of us who enjoy the challenge of a complex problem, PCOS research has a lot to offer. I hope the material in this chapter helps inspire research projects that lead to useful findings and practical applications. There are questions that have very concrete implications: for example, is there a way of reducing androgenisation prenatally in a PCOS pregnancy? To answer such questions we need well-designed research to assess the levels of testosterone experienced by the fetus in a PCOS pregnancy. Such research must use an adequate sample size and assay, and sample serum from the umbilical arteries and vein separately. Other issues are of more theoretical interest: for example, is it generally true that in women the direct effects of testosterone are more positive (as seen with mental rotation ability and libido), and the indirect effects more negative (as seen in reaction to physical symptoms, hypoglycaemia, and prenatal androgenisation)? The answers remain to be seen, as we explore and accumulate more information regarding the various psychobiological pathways in PCOS.

References

Abbott, D. H., Dumesic, D. A., Eisner, J. R., Colman, R. J., & Kemnitz, J. W. (1998). Insights into the development of polycystic ovary syndrome (PCOS) from studies of prenatally androgenized female rhesus monkeys. *Trends in Endocrinology & Metabolism, 9*, 62–67.

Abbott, D. H., Dumesic, D. A., & Franks, S. (2002). Developmental origin of polycystic ovary syndrome—A hypothesis. *The Journal of Endocrinology, 174*, 1–5.

Abbott, D. H., Dumesic, D. A., & Levine, J. E. (2019). Hyperandrogenic origins of polycystic ovary syndrome–implications for pathophysiology and therapy. *Expert Review of Endocrinology and Metabolism, 14*(2), 131–143.

Altuntas, Y., Bilir, M., Ucak, S., & Gundogdu, S. (2005). Reactive hypoglycemia in lean young women with PCOS and correlations with insulin sensitivity and with beta cell function. *European Journal of Obstetrics & Gynecology and Reproductive Biology, 119*(2), 198–205.

Anderson, H., Fogel, N., Grebe, S. K., Singh, R. J., Taylor, R. L., & Dunaif, A. (2010). Infants of women with polycystic ovary syndrome have lower cord blood androstenedione and estradiol levels. *The Journal of Clinical Endocrinology & Metabolism, 95*(5), 2180–2186.

Annagür, B. B., Tazegül, A., Uguz, F., Kerimoglu, Ö. S., Tekinarslan, E., & Celik, Ç. (2013). Biological correlates of major depression and generalized anxiety disorder in women with polycystic ovary syndrome. *Journal of Psychosomatic Research, 74*(3), 244–247.

Bammann, B. L., Coulam, C. B., & Jiang, N. S. (1980). Total and free testosterone during pregnancy. *American Journal of Obstetrics & Gynecology, 137*(3), 293–298.

Barry, J. A. (2011). *Exploration of biological causes of psychological problems in polycystic ovary syndrome (PCOS)*. Doctoral dissertation, City University London.

Barry, J. A., & Owens, R. (2019). From fetuses to boys to men: the impact of testosterone on male lifespan development. In *The Palgrave handbook of male psychology and mental health* (pp. 3–24). Cham: Palgrave Macmillan.

Barry, J. A., Kay, A. R., Navaratnarajah, R., Iqbal, S., Bamfo, J. E., David, A. L., … Hardiman, P. J. (2010). Umbilical vein testosterone in female infants born to mothers with polycystic ovary syndrome is elevated to male levels. *Journal of Obstetrics and Gynaecology, 1*, 444–446.

Barry, J. A., Bouloux, P., & Hardiman, P. J. (2011a). The impact of eating behavior on psychological symptoms typical of reactive hypoglycemia. A pilot study comparing women with polycystic ovary syndrome to controls. *Appetite, 57*, 73–76.

Barry, J. A., Hardiman, P. J., Saxby, B. K., & Kuczmierczyk, A. (2011b). Testosterone and mood dysfunction in women with polycystic ovarian syndrome compared to subfertile controls. *Journal of Psychosomatic Obstetrics and Gynecology, 32*, 104–111.

Barry, J. A., Hardiman, P. J., Siddiqui, M. R., & Thomas, M. (2011c). Meta-analysis of sex difference in testosterone levels in umbilical cord blood. *Journal of Obstetrics and Gynaecology, 31*(8), 697–702.

Barry, J. A., Kuczmierczyk, A. R., & Hardiman, P. J. (2011d). Anxiety and depression in polycystic ovary syndrome: A systematic review and meta-analysis. *Human Reproduction, 26*(9), 2442–2451.

Barry, J. A., Parekh, H. S. K., & Hardiman, P. J. (2013). Visual-spatial cognition in women with polycystic ovarian syndrome: The role of androgens. *Human Reproduction, 28*(10), 2832–2837.

Barry, J. A., Qu, F., & Hardiman, P. J. (2018). An exploration of the hypothesis that testosterone is implicated in the psychological functioning of women with polycystic ovary syndrome (PCOS). *Medical Hypotheses, 110*, 42–45.

Beck-Peccoz, P., Padmanabhan, V., Baggiani, A. M., Cortelazzi, D., Buscaglia, M., Medri, G., … Beitins, I. Z. (1991). Maturation of hypothalamic–pituitary–gonadal function in normal human fetuses: Circulating levels of gonadotropins, their common alpha-subunit and free testosterone, and discrepancy between immunological and biological activities of circulating follicle-stimulating hormone. *The Journal of Clinical Endocrinology & Metabolism, 73*, 525–532.

Benítez, R., Sir-Petermann, T., Palomino, A., Angel, B., Maliqueo, M., Pérez, F., & Calvillán, M. (2001). Prevalence of metabolic disorders among family members of patients with polycystic ovary syndrome. *Revista médica de Chile, 129*(7), 707–712. Spanish.

Bertalan, R., Csabay, L., Blazovics, A., Rigo, J., Jr., Varga, I., Halasz, Z., … Racz, K. (2007). Maternal hyperandrogenism beginning from early pregnancy and progressing until delivery does not produce virilization of a female newborn. *Gynecological Endocrinology, 23*(10), 581–583.

Birch, R. A., Padmanabhan, V., Foster, D. L., Unsworth, W. P., & Robinson, J. E. (2003). Prenatal programming of reproductive neuroendocrine function: Fetal androgen exposure produces progressive disruption of reproductive cycles in sheep. *Endocrinology, 144*, 1426–1434.

Bolton, N. J., Tapanainen, J., Koivisto, M., & Vihko, R. (1989). Circulating sex hormone-binding globulin and testosterone in newborns and infants. *Clinical Endocrinology (Oxford), 31*(2), 201–207.

Bramble, M. S., Roach, L., Lipson, A., Vashist, N., Eskin, A., Ngun, T., … Vilain, E. (2016). Sex-specific effects of testosterone on the sexually dimorphic transcriptome and epigenome of embryonic neural stem/progenitor cells. *Scientific Reports, 6*, 36916.

Brand-Miller, J., Farid, N. R., & Marsh, K. (2004). *The low GI guide to managing PCOS*. London: Hodder & Stoughton.

Carlsen, S. M., & Vanky, E. (2010). Metformin influence on hormone levels at birth, in PCOS mothers and their newborns. *Human Reproduction, 25*(3), 786–790.

Cefalu, W. T., & Pardridge, W. M. (2006). Restrictive transport of a lipid-soluble peptide (cyclosporin) through the blood–brain barrier. *Journal of Neurochemistry, 45*(6), 1954–1956.

Clarke, I. J., Scaramuzzi, R. J., & Short, R. V. (1977). Ovulation in prenatally androgenized ewes. *The Journal of Endocrinology, 73*, 385–389.

Conte, F. A., Grumbach, M. M., Ito, Y., Fisher, C. R., & Simpson, E. R. (1994). A syndrome of female pseudohermaphrodism, hypergonadotropic hypogonadism, and multicystic ovaries associated with missense mutations in the gene encoding aromatase (P450arom). *The Journal of Clinical Endocrinology & Metabolism, 78*(6), 1287–1292.

Cresswell, J. L., Barker, D. J., Osmond, C., Egger, P., Phillips, D. I., & Fraser, R. B. (1997). Fetal growth, length of gestation, and polycystic ovaries in adult life. *Lancet, 350*(9085), 1131–1135.

de Zegher, F., & Ibáñez, L. (2006). Prenatal growth restraint followed by catch-up of weight: A hyperinsulinemic pathway to polycystic ovary syndrome. *Fertility and Sterility, 86*, S4–S5.

Defreyne, J., Kreukels, B., T'Sjoen, G., Stahporsius, A., Den Heijer, M., Heylens, G., & Elaut, E. (2019). No correlation between serum testosterone levels and state-level anger intensity in transgender people: Results from the European network for the investigation of gender incongruence. *Hormones and Behavior, 110*, 29–39.

Demisch, K., Grant, J. K., & Black, W. (1968). Plasma testosterone in woman in late pregnancy and after delivery. *Journal of Endocrinology, 42*(3), 477–481.

Dumesic, D. A., Abbott, D. H., & Padmanabhan, V. (2007). Polycystic ovary syndrome and its developmental origins. *Reviews in Endocrine & Metabolic Disorders, 8*, 127–141.

Embryology.ch. (2007). Placental blood circulation. In *Human embryology*. Retrieved May 14, 2019, from http://www.embryology.ch/anglais/fplacenta/circulplac01.html.

Enjezab, B., Eftekhar, M., & Ghadiri-Anari, A. (2017). Association between severity of depression and clinico-biochemical markers of polycystic ovary syndrome. *Electronic Physician, 9*(11), 5820.

Filippou, P., & Homburg, R. (2017). Is foetal hyperexposure to androgens a cause of PCOS? *Human Reproduction Update, 23*(4), 421–432.

Foecking, E. M., Szabo, M., Schwartz, N. B., & Levine, J. F. (2005). Neuroendocrine consequences of prenatal androgen exposure in the female rat: Absence of luteinizing hormone surges, suppression of progesterone receptor gene expression, and acceleration of the gonadotropin-releasing hormone pulse generator. *Biology of Reproduction, 72*, 1475–1483.

Foulk, R. A., Martin, M. C., Jerkins, G. L., & Laros, R. K. (1997). Hyperreactio luteinalis differentiated from severe ovarian hyperstimulation syndrome in a spontaneously conceived pregnancy. *American Journal of Obstetrics and Gynecology, 176*(6), 1300–1302. discussion 1302–1304.

Franks, S., Mccarthy, M. I., & Hardy, K. (2006). Development of polycystic ovary syndrome: Involvement of genetic and environmental factors. *International Journal of Andrology, 29*(1), 278–285.

Furuhashi, N., Fukaya, T., Kono, H., Tachibana, Y., Shinkawa, O., & Takahashi, T. (1981). Sex differences in correlation coefficient among the cord serum levels of LH-hCG, beta-hCG, FSH, estradiol cortisol and testosterone (author's transl). *Nippon Sanka Fujinka Gakkai Zasshi, 33*(11), 1905–1909. Japanese.

Gold, A. E., MacLeod, K. M., Frier, B. M., & Deary, I. J. (1995). Changes in mood during acute hypoglycemia in healthy participants. *Journal of Personality and Social Psychology, 68*(3), 498.

Greenwood, E. A., Pasch, L. A., Cedars, M. I., Legro, R. S., Huddleston, H. G., Network, H. D. R. M., & Eunice Kennedy Shriver National Institute of

Child Health. (2018). Association among depression, symptom experience, and quality of life in polycystic ovary syndrome. *American Journal of Obstetrics and Gynecology, 219*(3), 279.e1.

Grumbach, M. M., & Ducharme, J. R. (1960). The effects of androgens on fetal sexual development: Androgen-induced female pseudohermaphrodism. *Fertility and Sterility, 11*, 157–180.

Hashimoto, D. M., Schmid, J., Martins, F. M., Fonseca, A. M., Andrade, L. H. B., Kirchengast, S., & Eggers, S. (2003). The impact of the weight status on subjective symptomatology of the polycystic ovary syndrome: A cross-cultural comparison between Brazilian and Austrian women. *Anthropologischer Anzeiger*, 297–310.

Hines, M. (2004). *Brain gender*. New York: Oxford University Press.

Hines, M. (2009). Gonadal hormones and sexual differentiation of human brain and behavior. In D. W. Pfaff (Ed.), *Hormones, brain and behavior* (2nd ed., pp. 1869–1909). New York: Academic Press.

Hollinrake, E., Abreu, A., Maifeld, M., Van Voorhis, B. J., & Dokras, A. (2007). Increased risk of depressive disorders in women with polycystic ovary syndrome. *Fertility and Sterility, 87*, 1369–1376.

Holt, H. B., Medbak, S., Kirk, D., Guirgis, R., Hughes, I., Cummings, M. H., & Meeking, D. R. (2005). Recurrent severe hyperandrogenism during pregnancy: A case report. *Journal of Clinical Pathology, 58*(4), 439–442.

Kasim-Karakas, S. E., Cunningham, W. M., & Tsodikov, A. (2007). Relation of nutrients and hormones in polycystic ovary syndrome. *American Journal of Clinical Nutrition, 85*, 688–694.

Klimczak, D., Szlendak-Sauer, K., & Radowicki, S. (2015). Depression in relation to biochemical parameters and age in women with polycystic ovary syndrome. *European Journal of Obstetrics & Gynecology and Reproductive Biology, 184*, 43–47.

Legro, R. S., Schlaff, W. D., Diamond, M. P., Coutifaris, C., Casson, P. R., Brzyski, R. G., ... Ohl, D. (2010). Total testosterone assays in women with polycystic ovary syndrome: Precision and correlation with hirsutism. *The Journal of Clinical Endocrinology & Metabolism, 95*(12), 5305–5313.

Leowattana, W. (2004). DHEAS as a new diagnostic tool. *Clinica Chimica Acta, 341*(1–2), 1–15.

Maccoby, E. E., Doering, C. H., Jacklin, C. N., & Kraemer, H. (1979). Concentrations of sex hormones in umbilical-cord blood: Their relation to sex and birth order of infants. *Child Development, 50*(3), 632–642.

Maliqueo, M., Lara, H. E., Sánchez, F., Echiburú, B., Crisosto, N., & Sir-Petermann, T. (2013). Placental steroidogenesis in pregnant women with polycystic ovary syndrome. *European Journal of Obstetrics & Gynecology and Reproductive Biology, 166*(2), 151–155.

Manikkam, M., Steckler, T. L., Welch, K. B., Inskeep, E. K., & Padmanabhan, V. (2006). Fetal programming: Prenatal testosterone treatment leads to follicular persistence/luteal defects; partial restoration of ovarian function by cyclic progesterone treatment. *Endocrinology, 147*(4), 1997–2007.

Mathur, R. S., Landgrebe, S., Moody, L. O., Powell, S., & Williamson, H. O. (1980). Plasma steroid concentrations in maternal and umbilical circulation after spontaneous onset of labor. *The Journal of Clinical Endocrinology and Metabolism, 51*(6), 1235–1238.

McKenna, T. J., & Cunningham, S. K. (1995). Adrenal androgen production in polycystic ovary syndrome. *European Journal of Endocrinology, 133*(4), 383–389.

Milutinović, D. V., Macut, D., Božić, I., Nestorov, J., Damjanović, S., & Matić, G. (2011). Hypothalamic-pituitary-adrenocortical axis hypersensitivity and glucocorticoid receptor expression and function in women with polycystic ovary syndrome. *Experimental and Clinical Endocrinology & Diabetes, 119*(10), 636–643.

Moran, C., Reyna, R., Boots, L. S., & Azziz, R. (2004). Adrenocortical hyper-responsiveness to corticotropin in polycystic ovary syndrome patients with adrenal androgen excess. *Fertility and Sterility, 81*(1), 126–131.

Nestler, J. E. (1987). Modulation of aromatase and P450 cholesterol side-chain cleavage enzyme activities of human placental cytotrophoblasts by insulin and insulin-like growth factor I. *Endocrinology, 121*(5), 1845–1852.

Ong, K. K., Ahmed, M. L., Emmett, P. M., Preece, M. A., & Dunger, D. B. (2000). Association between postnatal catch-up growth and obesity in childhood: Prospective cohort study. *BMJ, 320*(7240), 967–971. Erratum in: BMJ 2000 May 6;320(7244):1244.

Papalou, O., & Diamanti-Kandarakis, E. (2017). The role of stress in PCOS. *Expert Review of Endocrinology & Metabolism, 12*(1), 87–95.

Rahiminejad, M. E., Moaddab, A., Rabiee, S., Esna-Ashari, F., Borzouei, S., & Hosseini, S. M. (2014). The relationship between clinicobiochemical markers and depression in women with polycystic ovary syndrome. *Iranian Journal of Reproductive Medicine, 12*(12), 811.

Reiche, E. M. V., Nunes, S. O. V., & Morimoto, H. K. (2004). Stress, depression, the immune system, and cancer. *The Lancet Oncology, 5*(10), 617–625.

Resko, J. A., & Ellinwood, W. E. (1984). Sexual differentiation of the brain of primates. In M. Serio, M. Motta, M. Zanisi, & L. Martini (Eds.), *Sexual differentiation: Basic and clinical aspects* (pp. 169–181). New York: Raven Press.

Resko, J. A., Buhl, A. E., & Phoenix, C. H. (1987). Treatment of pregnant rhesus macaques with testosterone propionate: Observations on its fate in the fetus. *Biology of Reproduction, 37*, 1185–1191.

Roselli, C. F. (2007). Brain aromatase: Roles in reproduction and neuroprotection. *The Journal of Steroid Biochemistry and Molecular Biology, 106*(1–5), 143–150.

Shepard, R. N., & Metzler, J. (1971). Mental rotation of three-dimensional objects. *Science, 171*(3972), 701–703.

Sir-Petermann, T., Hitchsfeld, C., Maliqueo, M., Codner, E., Echiburú, B., Gazitúa, R., ... Cassorla, F. (2005). Birth weight in offspring of mothers with polycystic ovarian syndrome. *Human Reproduction, 20*(8), 2122–2126. Epub 2005 Mar 31.

Smail, P. J., Reyes, F. I., Winter, J. S. D., & Faiman, C. (1981). The fetal hormonal environment and its effect on the morphogenesis of the genital system. In S. J. Kogan & E. S. E. Hafez (Eds.), *Pediatric andrology* (pp. 9–19). The Hague: Martinus Nijhoff.

Soderlund, D., Canto, P., Carranza-Lira, S., & Mendez, J. P. (2005). No evidence of mutations in the P450 aromatase gene in patients with polycystic ovary syndrome. *Human Reproduction, 20*(4), 965–969.

Stanley, T., & Misra, M. (2008). Polycystic ovary syndrome in obese adolescents. *Current Opinion in Endocrinology, Diabetes and Obesity, 15*, 30–36.

Sullivan, S. D., & Moenter, S. M. (2004). Prenatal androgens alter GABAergic drive to gonadotropin-releasing hormone neurons: Implications for a common fertility disorder. *Proceedings of the National Academy of Sciences, 101*(18), 7129–7134.

Tata, B., Mimouni, N. E. H., Barbotin, A. L., Malone, S. A., Loyens, A., Pigny, P., ... Dal Bello, F. (2018). Elevated prenatal anti-Müllerian hormone reprograms the fetus and induces polycystic ovary syndrome in adulthood. *Nature Medicine, 24*(6), 834.

Thayer, R. E. (1989). *The biopsychology of mood and arousal.* London: Oxford University Press.

Troisi, R., Potischman, N., Roberts, J. M., Harger, G., Markovic, N., Cole, B., ... Hoover, R. N. (2003a). Correlation of serum hormone concentrations in maternal and umbilical cord samples. *Cancer Epidemiology Biomarkers and Prevention, 12*(5), 452–456.

Troisi, R., Potischman, N., Roberts, J., Siiteri, P., Daftary, A., Sims, C., & Hoover, R. N. (2003b). Associations of maternal and umbilical cord hormone concentrations with maternal, gestational and neonatal factors (United States). *Cancer Causes Control, 14*(4), 347–355.

van de Beek, C., Thijssen, J. H., Cohen-Kettenis, P. T., van Goozen, S. H., & Buitelaar, J. K. (2004). Relationships between sex hormones assessed in amniotic fluid, and maternal and umbilical cord serum: What is the best source of information to investigate the effects of fetal hormonal exposure? *Hormones and Behavior, 46*(5), 663–669.

Vottero, A., Stratakis, C. A., Ghizzoni, L., Longui, C. A., Karl, M., & Chrousos, G. P. (1999). Androgen receptor-mediated hypersensitivity to androgens in women with nonhyperandrogenic hirsutism: Skewing of X-chromosome inactivation. *The Journal of Clinical Endocrinology & Metabolism, 84*(3), 1091–1095.

Xita, N., Georgiou, I., Lazaros, L., Psofaki, V., Kolios, G., & Tsatsoulis, A. (2008). The synergistic effect of sex hormone-binding globulin and aromatase genes on polycystic ovary syndrome phenotype. *European Journal of Endocrinolog, 158*(6), 861–865.

Zharikova, O. L., Deshmukh, S. V., Nanovskaya, T. N., Hankins, G. D., & Ahmed, M. S. (2006). The effect of methadone and buprenorphine on human placental aromatase. *Biochemical Pharmacology, 71*(8), 1255–1264. Epub 2006 Feb 7.

8

Treatments for Improving Psychological Health in PCOS

Abstract For clinical psychologists and other psychological therapists, this chapter is likely to be the one of most interest. After all, for many people, the value of a science of psychology is most clearly demonstrated if something of clinical value comes of it. Although there is lots of room for the development of psychological interventions in this field, this chapter reveals that the few studies that have been done are so far innovative and show promise. This chapter explores how CBT and relaxation therapies can be adapted for women with PCOS, and how other interventions—medication, weight loss, and treating PCOS symptoms—can also be used to improve mental health in PCOS.

Keywords Cognitive behavioural therapy • Mindfulness • Relaxation • Guided imagery • Weight loss

Introduction

Stapinska-Syniec et al. (2018) found 64% (160 of 250) of women with PCOS said that psychological consultation should be offered to all women with PCOS. At the present time, those women would be

© The Author(s) 2019
J. A. Barry, *Psychological Aspects of Polycystic Ovary Syndrome*,
https://doi.org/10.1007/978-3-030-30290-0_8

disappointed that the provision of psychological services for women with PCOS falls well below 64%, and is much closer to 0%. We have seen in previous chapters that stress is a serious issue in PCOS, so it is ironic that healthcare provision—or rather, the lack thereof—actually contributes to this stress. Even for the medical aspects of PCOS, healthcare professionals may not immediately recognise the symptoms of PCOS in new patients, and treatment options are likely to be limited. The patient's initial contact with healthcare and diagnosis is a vulnerable time for women with PCOS, and has been described as a physical and 'emotional roller-coaster ride' (Gibson-Helm et al. 2017). Quicker diagnosis and quicker referral to good treatment options is needed.

The lack of mental health services provision for women with PCOS isn't because of a lack of available funding, or lack of therapists; it reflects: (a) the fact that the psychological aspects of PCOS are not on the radar of most professional psychologists and other psychological therapists, and (b) the cause of the increased risk of depression and anxiety in PCOS is not generally understood (Cooney and Dokras 2017). Furthermore, as will be seen in this chapter, there is very little research on what to offer women with PCOS for mental health issues.

It could be argued there are established interventions for some of the symptoms of PCOS, and women with PCOS can simply be referred there. For example, many psychological therapists who specialise in treating eating disorders can improve body image in PCOS, and improvements are possible even without weight loss or other physical changes (Thompson et al. 1999). This might be a good start, but evidence-based psychological interventions specifically for the complex issues around PCOS are needed.

PCOS is a heterogeneous condition, and we should be cautious about making too many assumptions about what an individual client wants. For example, some women will be more concerned about anxiety related to hirsutism, and others concerned with depression related to obesity. Also, age is a factor: younger women might want to have more healthy skin, but older women might be more concerned about fertility. As a general rule, health professionals should find out what it is that the PCOS client wants (Sullivan 2017), but they should also bear in mind that although younger women usually don't want to start a family immediately, as they get older, they might change their mind, sometimes quite suddenly (see also Chap. 6 on fertility). Difficulties related to pregnancy (conception, miscarriage, abnormalities), which increase as healthy women grow older, may be especially problematic for women with PCOS. The responsible health professional will, with sensitivity, make the younger woman with PCOS aware of the risks that she faces. Researchers and policymakers should be busy in the background trying to ensure that these risks are reduced in the coming decades, so that the adolescent with PCOS today has a better reproductive future than those who have gone before.

Culture is also a factor. Obesity is an issue for women in most cultures, but there are interesting cross-cultural differences. For example, for Brazilian women with PCOS, fertility problems had a worse QoL impact than weight issues. However having an 'apple shaped' body (gaining weight around the abdomen) rather than 'pear shaped' obesity (gaining weight around the hips) is considered unattractive in many cultures (Brown 1991).

Due to the very limited amount of research on interventions to help psychological symptoms of PCOS, in the present chapter some of the material will be extrapolating from research in non-PCOS women in order to suggest sensible ways of developing treatment for women with PCOS. I hope that by the time it comes to a second edition of this book, more research on psychological interventions for PCOS will have been conducted so that more evidence-based information can be shared.

In this chapter I will focus on three approaches to helping with the psychological aspects of PCOS. The first is to use standard psychological therapies. The second is to use relaxation interventions. The third is to improve psychological well-being in PCOS by improving the symptoms of PCOS. After this, psychological interventions for weight loss will be explored.

Cognitive Behavioural Therapy (CBT)

CBT can be described as 'a talking therapy that can help you manage your problems by changing the way you think and behave. It's most commonly used to treat anxiety and depression, but can be useful for other mental and physical health problems. CBT is based on the concept that your thoughts, feelings, physical sensations and actions are interconnected, and that negative thoughts and feelings can trap you in a vicious cycle' (NHS 2019). Elizabeth et al. (2009) suggest that CBT might help women with PCOS. Based on interventions with non-PCOS women with chronic problems, Elizabeth et al. suggest that a six-step behavioural change process to improve 'change resilience' might help women with PCOS too.

CBT is perhaps the most ubiquitous of all the psychological therapies practised by psychologists today, and has perhaps the largest evidence base. This being the case, it is remarkable that our knowledge of the benefits of CBT for women with PCOS is—to say the least—scant. A *Google Scholar* search for academic publications since the year 2000 with 'cognitive behavioural therapy' in the title, finds over 2000 examples of the application of CBT to a wide variety of conditions, but to date, only four studies—one of them a case study of a single patient—exist on the use of CBT for PCOS. I outline these four pioneering studies below.

A case study by Correa et al. (2015) found that a workbook based on CBT helped a young woman with PCOS with her anxiety, depression, psychosocial problems, eating habits, and a significant loss in weight. Rofey et al. (2009) conducted the first study of CBT for PCOS. This was a good quality pilot study of CBT with 12 adolescents (aged 12–18) with PCOS, obesity, and mild depression. Participants were recruited from Pittsburg Hospital and were excluded if they had an existing serious psychiatric condition or were on antidepressant medication. If they were seeing a therapist for current depression they could join the study, provided they suspended their treatment for the duration of the study. Participants filled in The Children's Depression Inventory (CDI), and then followed the Primary and Secondary Control Enhancement Training (PASCET-PI-2) course, which addresses control issues, coping, and family issues around dealing with emotions and illness. It was found that 8 weekly sessions (see text box) significantly improved depression scores ($p < 0.01$) and weight (mean 104 kg to 93 kg; $p < 0.05$). Although a good quality trial, there are limitations inherent to pilot studies of this kind, such as the small sample size and lack of a control group. Also we can't be sure how well the findings with such a young sample, completing child-specific questionnaires, generalises to adult women with PCOS filling the BDI or HADS. Nonetheless, the study by Rofey et al. is a landmark in PCOS and sets the standard for others to build upon.

> Rofey et al. (2009) CBT programme for adolescents with PCOS. All sessions started with a weigh-in, then 45–60 minutes of CBT, then 20 minutes of physical exercise.
>
> **Session 1.** Psychoeducation about physical illness, depression, and CBT; lifestyle change. Additional 60 minutes of similar work with family.
>
> **Session 2.** Problem-solving, coping; sleep; lifestyle diary, understanding food.
>
> **Session 3.** Enjoying physical activity; social skills; goal setting; understanding hunger.
>
> **Session 4.** Relaxation; planning enjoyable events and healthy meals. Additional 60 minutes with family regarding progress, expressing emotion, and a game to reduce expressed emotion.
>
> **Session 5.** Positivity, motivation, body image; lifestyle goals; decreasing sedentary behaviour.
>
> **Session 6.** Cognitive distortions, self-esteem; review of body image diary and sleep.
>
> **Session 7.** Cognitive distortions; coping (e.g. with bullying).
>
> **Session 8.** Reframing; social support; review of skills gained; *'lapse isn't relapse'*; scheduling booster sessions. Additional 60 minutes with family regarding progress and reinforcing skills.

Although Rofey et al. (2009) stated that 'This study lays the groundwork for future randomized comparison studies assessing the effectiveness of CBT in treating obesity and depression' (Rofey et al. 2009, p. 160), it is disappointing that a decade later, only two published studies have done so. Abdollahi (2016) conducted an RCT of 74 women with PCOS to either eight weekly sessions of group CBT or no-treatment control. Women newly diagnosed with PCOS, aged between 18 and 35 were recruited from various gynaecology clinics in Iran. They excluded from the study women with severe depression scores (BDI > 29) and those on psychiatric medication. CBT included psychoeducation on PCOS, relaxation techniques (including breathing and visualisation techniques), and the practice of learnings between each session. There were no significant differences in demographic variables. At baseline, both groups showed, on average, minor depression. The CBT group mean BDI was statistically significantly higher at baseline that in the control group (16.4 vs 13.7; $p < 0.014$), which is not ideal, but the more important finding was that the 4 weeks post-treatment the BDI scores had improved to a clinical and statistically significant degree in the CBT group (4.5 vs 16.5). After the intervention, the mean $\pm$ SD BMI scores changed very little as a result of the intervention (pre-CBT = 27.6 $\pm$ 5.9; post-CBT 27.3 $\pm$ 5.4), though the very short follow-up period (4 weeks) is not long enough to see much change in BMI (three months is a more reasonable minimum follow-up period for psychological interventions). Also, a no-treatment control group is probably the least preferable type of control group, because it sets the bar minimally low against the treatment group. For example, the treatment group may improve due a placebo effect (expectations regarding the intervention), or a Hawthorne effect (response to receiving the extra attention of being in a study). For this reason, a having 'treatment as usual' control group (TAU) is preferable, because this gives a recognised standard against which the experimental group changes can be measured. A suitable TAU for PCOS research might be a generic version of CBT without any specific reference to PCOS (e.g. no psychoeducational aspect). Also preferable to a no-treatment group is a 'waiting list' control group; participants in this group give scores on the outcome measures at the same measurement occasions as the experimental group, and have the benefit of knowing that they are going to receive the treatment once the experimental group has completed theirs.

Cooney et al. (2018) conducted a pilot study, randomising women with PCOS, who were also overweight or obese, and were depressed, either to 8 weeks of CBT + 16 weeks of lifestyle counselling ($n = 7$) or just 16 weeks of lifestyle counselling ($n = 8$). Lifestyle counselling consisted of 30 minutes per week with a trained counsellor, for training in diet and exercise skills and strategies. The CBT group additionally had 30 minutes per week with a clinical psychologist trained in CBT. The CBT included dealing with automatic thoughts and cognitive distortions, activity scheduling, and homework, all based on *The Brief Cognitive Therapy Manual* (Cully and Teten 2008). At the end of week 16, the CBT group had lost more weight than the other group (3.2 kg vs 1.8 kg; $p < 0.08$), had improved WHR (0.05 vs 0.0; $p < 0.049$), greater improvement in PCOSQ for hirsutism (3.7 vs 1.2 points; $p < 0.049$), and greater reduction in total cholesterol (-19 vs $+3$ mg/dL; $p < 0.03$). Some other measures improved at week 8 (systolic blood pressure, overall PCOSQ, and PCOSQ for menstrual functioning), but did not remain significantly improved at week 16. This study used an impressive range of outcomes (including markers of inflammation not mentioned here), and although the sample size was small, this was mainly due to the 50% dropout over the course of the study, particularly from the CBT group early in the study, mainly due to time commitment issues experienced by participants.

This well-conducted study highlights the problems caused by dropout in longitudinal studies, and the need to find ways to reduce it (e.g. by identifying motivational weaknesses at baseline) where possible. Of relevance to motivation is the study by Hopkins et al. (2019) of 23 adolescents (aged 13–18) with PCOS, who found that the top three stressors they experienced in relation to PCOS were weight, periods, and future infertility. Although the aim of the study was not about dropout, of relevance to this issue was ambivalence expressed over how much control participants had over weight, with one participant saying: 'I'll lose like 5 or 10 pounds, then I gain 20 back' (Hopkins et al. 2019, p. 194). It might be useful, therefore, for a future study to find out the benefits to participants in longitudinal interventions of being given a realistic but robust sense of control over their weight loss.

Relaxation and Guided Imagery

Another approach to helping with psychological issues in PCOS is to use relaxation. Relaxation therapy can be delivered either as a method of simply inducing relaxation, or can be delivered with the addition of CBT or guided imagery. Guided imagery typically asks the participant to imagine themselves experiencing pleasant situations (e.g. relaxing on a beach) and/

or achieving relevant goals (e.g. enjoying exercise). However, because moderate to severe anxiety effects around 45% of women with PCOS (Chap. 3), and stress can increase adrenal androgen production (Chap. 7), relaxation is of special relevance for women with PCOS. We have seen from Chap. 7 that one of the pathways in PCOS is from the endocrine system to the mind (Fig. 7.2, yellow arrows), and that it is possible that this pathway can be used in the other direction—from the mind to the endocrine system (Fig. 7.3, yellow arrow). Evidence suggests that relaxation techniques can reduce hypothalamic-pituitary axis (HPA) activity, alleviate anxiety and depression, and improve QoL and well-being (Deng and Cassileth 2005). As stated by Farrell and Antoni: 'addressing psychological disturbances can reduce or alleviate physical symptoms of PCOS through behavioral pathways and physiological pathways' (Farrell and Antoni 2010, p. 1565).

A pioneering study in the use of relaxation by Stefanaki et al. (2015) was the first to demonstrate that a psychological intervention—mindfulness training—could reduce adrenal gland activity in women with PCOS. Stefanaki et al. randomised 46 women with PCOS to either 8 weeks of mindfulness training or no-treatment control group. After allocation to the intervention or control condition, participants in the intervention group were trained (presumably for about 30 minutes) in the stress-management programme, which included mindfulness breathing and diaphragmatic breathing exercises. This was subsequently delivered by audio compact disc (CD) for 30 minutes for 8 weeks, usually before bedtime. Each week the participant could opt to also discuss their progress with the principal investigator for 30 minutes each week, in person or by phone. At the end of the study period, the intervention group scored better than the control group on several of the outcomes measured: depression was 4.3 ± 3.3 versus 17.2 ± 9.9 ($p < 0.01$); stress (but not anxiety) was 5.0 ± 4.0 versus 19.06 ± 9.6 ($p < 0.025$); total life satisfaction was 63.8 ± 9.7 versus 48.4 ± 7.9 ($p < 0.001$); waking cortisol levels 0.4 ± 0.1 versus 2.0 ± 0.8 ($p < 0.001$) and cortisol levels again 30 minutes after waking 0.8 ± 0.4 versus 2.5 ± 0.8 ($p < 0.025$). The scores in the intervention group also improved from baseline to post-study: depression 18.0 ± 8.0 to 4.34 ± 3.28 ($p < 0.01$); anxiety 12.0 ± 9.0 to 5.0 ± 4.0 ($p < 0.025$); all of the PCOSQ subscales (minimum $p < 0.006$); and general life satisfaction 25.0 ± 4.4 versus 27.0 ± 5.3 ($p < 0.03$). Interestingly, no significant differences were seen in the intervention group pre- and post- for cortisol levels nor stress scores despite the between-group differences on those measures.

This was an impressive study in assessing the impact of a relaxation training on not only psychological outcomes but also biochemical outcomes, and the breadth of outcomes measured (some are not mentioned above). There are a few minor points that I will highlight for the sake of helping with replications of this work. Firstly, all participants in the intervention group completed the study, whereas 8 of the controls (35%) dropped out. On a positive note, this suggests that the intervention group was engaging, but it also emphasises that a drawback of using a no-treatment control group is that those participants might lose motivation to continue with the study. One other issue is that it is best practice to include the baseline data of those who drop out in the analysis in order to take into account the possibility that those who dropped out were different to those who stayed in—for instance, possibly being significantly more depressed at baseline. This *intention-to-treat (ITT)* analysis can be done in various ways (e.g. the baseline-observation-carried-forward (BOCF) method), but no ITT was done in this study. This intervention, being on a CD, has the advantage of being easy to deliver and cost effective. Possible weaknesses were the use of a salivary cortisol measure, using salivettes and an electrochemiluminescence assay, which is a relatively rudimentary method of assessment. Also the impact of age was not taken fully into account, because the intervention group were on average 5 years younger than the control group (mean $\pm$ SD: 23.4 ± 4.62 vs 28.3 ± 4.62 years old). Although this is unlikely to have made a great deal of difference between groups (and no difference at all to the within-groups comparison), it would have been good to analyse the study data using ANCOVA, rather than a t-test, with age as a covariate.

Barry et al. (2017) conducted a study of relaxation with guided imagery aimed at decreasing androgen levels and improving mood (see text box). Thirteen women with PCOS underwent six weekly treatment sessions, with 12–15 minutes of diaphragmatic breathing, muscle relaxation, and guided imagery, with 30 minutes extra in session 1 (for introductions and information gathering), and session 6 (for discussing progress). Each week, guided imagery focused on a different aspect of PCOS, for example, if the participant had issues with body weight related to eating chocolate, the script would include phrases such as *'Imagine seeing yourself having much more control over how you think and feel about chocolate'.* There was one follow-up session 13 weeks after session 6. Anxiety and depression were measured on the HADS, and QoL on the PCOSQ. Hormone levels, including the adrenal androgens DHEAS and androstenedione, were assayed using liquid chromatography tandem mass spectrometry. There was a small but statistically significant reduction in DHEAS from before to after week 1 (3.6 ± 1.6 to 3.4 ± 1.4; $p < 0.044$) and from before to after week 6 (3.5 ± 1.4 to 3.3 ± 1.4; $p < 0.001$). From before to after week 6, there were also small but statistically significant reductions in androstenedione (3.9 ± 2.2 vs 3.5 ± 2.0; $p < 0.010$) and cortisol (200.0 ± 138.6 vs 160.2 ± 132.0; $p < 0.003$). From week 1 to week 6, there was a significant reduction in anxiety (11.1 ± 4.3 vs 8.6 ± 3.8; $p < 0.037$). There was a significant improvement in depression scores from week 1 to week 6 (6.4 ± 3.8 vs 4.3 ± 3.4; $p < 0.034$ [$n = 11$]) and from week 1 to follow-up (7.0 ± 3.9 vs 4.5 ± 3.3; $p < 0.011$ [$n = 8$]). There were no significant changes in free or total testosterone, nor in PCOSQ.

The hormonal findings demonstrate the validity of a psychobiological mechanism that is important to PCOS—the reduction of adrenal androgens using a non-pharmacological relaxation intervention. Although the changes were modest, we do not know how much clinical benefit there might be in such changes, because some people are quite sensitive to even small changes in androgen (Wang and Zane 2008). However, the intervention made no tangible impact on free or total testosterone levels, which could suggest that the testosterone being measured was of ovarian origin rather than a by-product of adrenal activity. This being the case, a future study might use guided imagery directed at reducing ovarian androgen production, or increasing ovarian estrogen production.

An interesting aspect of Barry et al. (2017) was that the longitudinal design allowed us to see that the effect of the intervention was cumulative over the 6 weeks, with the effects seen after week 1 becoming stronger at week 6. The longitudinal aspect shows that the physiological effect wore off after 13 weeks of no practice, though the effect on depression endured.

The improvements to anxiety and depression seen in this study were statistically significant. The change in anxiety scoring was also of marginal clinical significance, with average levels for the group falling from mild levels to almost normal levels. The depression levels fell significantly but only within the normal range, so the change for depression was not of clinical significance.

The weaknesses of this study are the small sample size and lack of control group. Two participants dropped out of the study after the first session: one participant did not appear to show any response to the treatment and the other said she didn't think that the programme was suitable for her. This shows that for relaxation therapy, like treatments of various kinds, one size does not fit all. But despite the small sample size and lack of control group, this pilot study has some merit. The assay used was the gold standard methodology for measuring androgen in women (liquid chromatography tandem mass spectrometry), so we can be relatively certain of the validity of the hormone levels found. Although lacking a control group, the repeated-measures design should not be underestimated, because it controls for many potential confounding variables (individual differences, medication use) otherwise seen when comparing different participants in different groups. The participants' use of medications (which was stable over the study period) of the kind typically seen in PCOS makes the findings generalisable to the average woman with PCOS.

The intervention we used was minimally complex in order that the programme could be relatively inexpensive to train researchers or medical staff in the technique and easy for other research groups to replicate. However it is interesting to compare this to the CD intervention of Stefanaki et al. (2015), which worked very well in improving several outcomes, but needed to be delivered every day for 30 minutes over 8 weeks (a total of 1680 minutes), instead of just once per week for 15 minutes for 6 weeks (a total of 150 minutes, including the longer first and sixth sessions). On the other hand, the CD would have been very convenient for participants to use, and they would not need to travel to see a therapist in order to receive the intervention. However it is likely that the effects found in Barry et al. (2017) could be intensified by extending the duration of the intervention (e.g. from 12–15 minutes to 20–30 minutes), and having more frequent sessions (e.g. two per week). It is likely that the delivery by an experienced and qualified practitioner (Noelia Leite in the Barry et al. study) would be more effective than delivery on a CD, not just because of the benefit of the more personal and human element of one-to-one interventions, but because the therapist can be sensitive to the participant's state from one session to another and adjust for this in how the session is delivered.

Although not measured as an outcome in either Stefanaki et al. (2015) or Barry et al. (2017), it is likely that participants would have experienced improved sleep, because this is a common benefit of relaxation therapies. This is important for many women with PCOS, because there is evidence that improvement of sleep quality can reduce obesity (Vgontzas 2008). Fernandez et al. (2018) suggest that 'Both immediate quality of life and longer-term health of women with PCOS are likely to benefit from diagnosis and management of sleep disorders as part of interdisciplinary health care' (Fernandez et al. 2018, p. 45).

Protocol for Barry et al. (2017).
Each session consists of about 12–15 minutes of diaphragmatic breathing, muscle relaxation, and guided imagery. There was an extra 30 minutes in the first and sixth session for introductions and conclusions.
Session 1: Overview of treatment plan, methods, and aims. History taking to identify main issues and more detailed explanation about the 6-week relaxation programme, identifying ideal self/situation.
Session 2: Exploration of level of self-esteem, and unhealthy behaviour related to it.
Session 3: Weight, low GI types of food, unhealthy eating patterns, food diary, and preferred pattern.
Session 4: Aggression and its main trigger(s) and preferred reaction.
Session 5: Exploration of skin-related issues and information treatment options (if necessary).
Session 6: Exploration of menstruation/fertility (or social skills, if menstruation/fertility was not an issue). Information and treatment options. End-of-treatment discussion.
Follow-up (approximately 13 weeks after Session 6): participants revisited the activities of weeks 1 and 6.

Suggested Techniques and Strategies for Treating Mood Issues in PCOS

Because of the lack of research on psychological treatment techniques and strategies for PCOS, I will make some suggestions in this section that might be useful. These are aimed at experienced practitioners of various schools of therapy, each of whom should use their own judgement and take sensible precautions in regards to how they see these fitting into their usual therapeutic approach and overall formulation of the issues.

Normalise Distress, While Being Mindful of Potential Suicide Risk

Much of the research into PCOS has been conducted at clinics, and consequently the findings are based on the least well and least happy cases (Ezeh et al. 2013). Women with PCOS who don't need much clinical care might form an unrealistically negative view of their prognosis, and it might be useful for the healthcare worker to assure their PCOS patient that things might not be as dire as are sometimes presented on the internet. 'Psychoeducation' regarding PCOS should include demystifying the term 'PCOS', which is difficult to understand, not least because patients don't need ovarian cysts to have a diagnosis of PCOS (see Chap. 1), and the term 'cyst' is often associated with cancer, or pus-filled growths, even though in PCOS, the 'cysts' are nothing like this.

Although one small study (Månsson et al. 2008) found a relatively high rate of suicide attempts in women with PCOS, the much larger study by Cesta et al. (2016) found that found that the odds of attempted suicide in women with PCOS were 41% higher than other women, in other words far less than double the risk. Any sign that a woman is suicidal should be treated in the usual way, taking into account their wider psychological formulation, and onward referral made if appropriate.

Psychological Techniques for Depression

We have already seen the impact of CBT interventions (e.g. Rofey et al. 2009) and relaxation interventions (e.g. Barry et al. 2017) for PCOS earlier. Both strategies appear promising for depression. We have seen in previous chapters that depression is probably caused by a depressiono-genic appraisal of the PCOS symptoms. Several avenues for treatment, which can be thought of as solution-focused, emotion-focused, or avoid-ant, might be taken. The following might be considered in tandem with treatment based on conventional guidelines:

1. *Remove the symptom*: e.g. weight loss. This solution-focused strategy makes sense, but can be costly, time-consuming, and difficult for women with PCOS who may be struggling against a lower basal meta-bolic rate and insulin resistance. We know that reducing BMI can improve hyperandrogenism and protect against CVD, so making healthy lifestyle changes is likely to be a good choice overall in the long term, due to psychological and potential physical benefits.
2. *Reduce anxiety about the symptom*: This is primarily an emotion-focused strategy, though is also potentially solution-focused. Using mindful-ness or relaxation can be effective, and relatively simple compared to CBT. It might also potentially reduce physiological symptoms through reduction of the production of adrenal androgen (Barry et al. 2017). A study of stress management in women with breast cancer found a reduction in testosterone (Cruess et al. 2001), but this study used a small sample and—to my knowledge—has not been replicated.

    Relaxation might also help reduce sleep disturbance. As noted in Chap. 3, poor sleep is associated with increased risk of type 2 diabetes, thereby increasing distressing PCOS symptoms (Fernandez et al. 2018).
3. *Put the symptom severity into perspective*: An emotion-focused approach. Methods such as REBT (David et al. 2018) can be used here to help the client to see the severity of their symptoms in relation to the sever-ity of other life experiences, for instance, 'Having facial hair isn't pleas-ant, but isn't the very worst possible thing that could happen to me'.
4. *Reframe the problem as an opportunity*: Avoidant strategy. For example, if a woman is infertile due to having PCOS, she might benefit by focussing on how it can mean she can dedicate her life to something

else meaningful to her—for example, a career, or being a fantastic aunt, or simply avoiding all of the stress and expense of raising children.

Some women with PCOS take this reframing a step further and are actively proud of their symptoms (e.g. the 'Armpits for August' campaign *https://armpitsforaugust.wordpress.com*). Although, the idea of rejecting social norms of female beauty might achieve a short-term lift in mood, it might be an uphill struggle with limited long term psychological benefit. This strategy risks leaving the woman with an outsider identity, which might be a burden in itself because of the energy required to constantly justify oneself, both to oneself and others.

Psychological Techniques for Anxiety

Although usually less the focus of attention than depression, anxiety is possibly a more complex and widespread issue in PCOS than depression. It is complex because of the issues discussed in Chap. 3, and relatively widespread because the meta-analysis by Cooney et al. (2017) found that the rates of moderate-to-severe anxiety are higher in women with PCOS than those for depression (44.9% vs 9.3%, according to my calculation in Chap. 3). Often anxiety and depression are comorbid, in which case whichever is more severe should be treated first (NICE 2018, p. 188).

We have already seen the impact of CBT interventions and relaxation interventions for PCOS earlier in this chapter. Both strategies appear promising for anxiety, particularly the relaxation strategies because of the impact on adrenal androgens. There is as yet no recommended treatment for anxiety for women with PCOS, but the techniques listed in the previous section for depression are likely to improve anxiety levels too. However the optimal treatment of anxiety may be different to treatment of depression, mainly because anxiety in PCOS might have a more direct physiological basis rooted in activation of the sympathetic nervous system (SNS).

Medication

Medication such as oral contraceptive pills and insulin-sensitising drugs can improve symptoms of PCOS. However, there are few studies of the psychological benefits of these medications, and even worse, there are no published studies to date evaluating the benefits of anti-depressants or anti-anxiety medications in PCOS (Cooney and Dokras 2017).

Oral contraceptives are a first-line intervention for PCOS. Although they can improve PCOS, the evidence is not consistent that they also improve psychology (see also section on OCPs in Chap. 6). For example, although one study has found an improvement in depression (Dokras et al. 2016), another found no impact on depression, despite improvements in hirsutism and menstrual functioning (Cinar et al. 2012). Although it has been found that 6 months of metformin improved psychiatric and physiological parameters in women with PCOS (Hahn et al. 2006), metformin does not seem to improve physiological responses to stress (Benson et al. 2009). This means that metformin is probably a better candidate for treatment of depression than anxiety, but more research is needed here.

A meta-analysis found that both orlistat and metformin can reduce weight in PCOS (Graff et al. 2016). Dokras et al. (2016) found orlistat or sibutramine combined with a stringent diet and exercise programme led to better weight loss than for a group randomised to taking only OCPs, though the study design makes it difficult to identify the contribution of weight loss medication to weight loss.

Medication may have side effects. For example, orlistat can help with weight loss but has unpleasant side effects (mainly, flatulence and oily stools). Metformin may also have mildly unpleasant gastrointestinal side effects in the first weeks of use (Fruzzetti et al. 2017).

Adrenal suppression, which could potentially be useful for anxiety, was once considered an effective treatment of PCOS symptoms (Kaltsas et al. 2003). However this treatment has lost popularity because patients are reluctant to take potent corticosteroids, even in low doses, when other medications (such as metformin) can be used in PCOS instead.

There is sometimes a dilemma over whether the patient should receive medication or talking therapy, but in many cases, the best approach is to use both (NHS 2016). In 'combination therapy', medication is used to lift mood to allow for appropriate cognitive restructuring to be done by the psychological therapist. It should be noted that 50 years of research on rational emotive behaviour therapy (REBT) has found that it similar benefits to medication in alleviating depression (David et al. 2018). Psychological therapies can be more cost effective and enduring than medication, and should be adjunctive to standard medical care in PCOS (Farrell and Antoni 2010). The Thessaloniki ESHRE/ASRM-Sponsored PCOS Consensus Workshop Group Consensus on infertility treatment related to PCOS (2008) suggests that counselling related to lifestyle changes should be delivered prior to pharmacologic interventions.

Improving Mood by Treating PCOS Symptoms

Several studies have used medical treatments for PCOS, and as part of the range of outcomes measured, assessed the impact on psychological factors such as depression, anxiety, and QoL. For example, Clayton et al. (2005) found that laser treatment for facial hirsutism improved HRQoL and HADS anxiety and depression scores in PCOS compared to controls, but no significant improvements in the QoL in the social or environmental domain were seen, nor self-esteem. However, as described in Chap. 3, QoL doesn't always correlate with objective symptoms.

One of the key issues in PCOS, both psychologically and physiologically, is obesity. The rest of this section will focus on what is called 'lifestyle modification' for weight control. In this chapter, surgical interventions (e.g. gastric band) won't be discussed, though they may have merit.

Lifestyle Modification: Diet and Exercise

Obesity is a key factor in PCOS for several reasons. Preventing obesity developing at puberty could prevent the development of PCOS. Once it is in place, obesity can cause insulin resistance and type 2 diabetes (Sam 2007), which in turn, can cause androgens to increase via decreased aromatase activity in adipose tissue (Wake et al. 2007), exacerbating the distressing symptoms of PCOS. Weight loss increases SHBG levels, thus reducing free testosterone levels and PCOS symptoms (Moran et al. 2003). Weight loss reduces the risk of diabetes and CVD, two chronic diseases associated with obesity and with PCOS. Therefore, tackling obesity is an obvious target for any healthcare worker dealing with PCOS. Even if weight loss is not achieved, exercise can improve ovulation, insulin resistance, and inflammation in PCOS (Farrell and Antoni 2010).

A review of QoL research found weight problems had the worst impact on women with PCOS (Jones et al. 2008). Higher BMI is correlated with worse QoL in women with PCOS (McCook et al. 2005; Hahn et al. 2005). Adolescents with PCOS have worse HRQoL for weight issues than healthy girls (Trent et al. 2005). Most studies find depression correlated with obesity in healthy women (Stunkard et al. 2003) and PCOS (Rasgon et al. 2003). This means that in terms of improving QoL in PCOS, reducing obesity is a key factor.

Binge Eating

As seen in Chap. 3, binge eating is around twice as common in PCOS than other women. Because changes in eating behaviour can impact the presence of polycystic ovaries (Himelein and Thatcher 2006), it is important to address any such disordered eating. In non-PCOS populations, CBT (Amianto et al. 2015) and mindfulness (Godfrey et al. 2015) have been found helpful in reducing food cravings related to binge eating. Future research should try such treatments with PCOS women.

Lifestyle Modification: Diet and Exercise

The first-line treatment in women with PCOS is lifestyle management, which usually means diet and exercise (Cooney and Dokras 2017). In the general population, a meta-analysis of 18 studies found that CBT induced an average weight loss of around 10 lbs (around 5 kg), most of which stayed off for two years (Kirsch et al. 1995). Kirsch et al. found that adding hypnotherapy to the CBT intervention doubled the effect on weight loss: the average weight loss was around 20 lbs (about 10 kg), all of which, on average, stayed off for two years. Cooney and Dokras (2017) list nine

RCTs of lifestyle management for PCOS. Their results generally showed benefits, though not always statistically significant, with some studies of lifestyle interventions for PCOS finding significant reductions in depression and/or anxiety. For example, Galletly et al. (2007) found a significant benefit of a high-protein/low-carbohydrate diet for depression, and Thomson et al. (2010) found a significant benefit of exercise on depression. So it seems that there is some benefit to anxiety and depression in losing weight, although it is not a consistent affect.

GPs (General Practitioners, or 'family doctors') are often the first person that a woman with PCOS consults regarding her symptoms. GPs are sometimes criticised for not knowing enough about PCOS or not being able to do offer practical solutions or help. Being told to improve their diet and exercise rather than being given a medical cure can be frustrating, but it can be good advice. Even getting out more into the sunshine can be beneficial: in a study of 114 women with PCOS, Naqvi et al. (2015) found that for those who were vitamin D deficient, their levels of vitamin D predicted their Personal Health Questionnaire (PHQ) scores.

Arasu et al. (2019) interviewed 15 general practitioners in Australia to find their opinions on the barriers and facilitators to weight and lifestyle management in women with PCOS. They found that every GP agreed that weight and lifestyle management is key to treating PCOS. The main barriers they reported were lack of funding for longer GP consultations, time constraints, patient motivation, and physical and financial accessibility to allied health professionals. The main facilitators were having a long-term doctor–patient relationship, the GP's communication skills, motivational interviewing, and allied health referrals. One thing to be learned was that GPs need to be able to refer more to psychologists who specialise in weight management, because without the funding to do so, GPs will rely on their own efforts at delivering counselling for lifestyle-related problems, much of which may be considered too generic for the specific needs of women with PCOS. GPs were inclined to refer mainly for fertility issues, but a greater use of referral to other experts might lead not only to greater weight loss success, but allow GPs more time to focus on other aspects of PCOS. This can be especially the case where the GP's efforts are undermined by what is seen as the poor motivation of the patient.

Arasu et al. (2019) is an interesting study, though future studies might see how their findings relate to a health belief model, such as the Integrative Model of Behaviour Prediction (IMBP, Fishbein et al. 2001), which specifies ways of measuring quantitatively patient barriers and facilitators, such as motivations. Jakubowski et al. (2012) conducted one of the few studies of psychological aspects of PCOS using a psychological model. Using the *stages of change* model (SOC; DiClemente and Prochaska 1982), they assessed the readiness of 40 adolescents with PCOS to lose weight. They found that, like many health behaviour models, the SOC did not predict weight loss. However the SOC did predict BMI change from the attitude of the adolescents' *parents*. This represented a shift in parents' attitudes to some, but not all, aspects of lifestyle change, specifically increasing fruit and vegetable intake and physical activity. This study demonstrates the importance of including the family in lifestyle changes in adolescents with PCOS as also done by Rofey et al. (2009).

Motivational Interviewing

Motivational interviewing (MI) is a brief method for identifying barriers and strengths in order to help patients to improve motivation to achieve a particular outcome. Moeller et al. (2019) randomised 37 obese women with PCOS to receive for six months either standard advice from their GP, or standard advice plus motivational interviewing. They found that the addition of MI improved depression scores, but not weight loss or QoL scores.

Stress and Weight Loss

Farrell and Antoni (2010) suggest it is possible that stress can both be an aspect of a maladaptive mindset, and also increase visceral fact via elevated cortisol, and that stress reduction could be an important adjunct to conventional treatment with insulin sensitisers. They also suggest that stress reduction might also help prevent the physiological damage stress causes through exacerbation of inflammation.

Exercise

Exercise improves ovulation in ~50% of women with PCOS (Harrison et al. 2010). In fact, even without weight loss, regular exercise improves ovulation and pregnancy rates (Huber-Buchholz et al. 1999). In a study of PCOS lasting 24 weeks, Palomba et al. (2008) found ovulation improved significantly more in the group taking exercise than a group dieting. Women with PCOS on an 8-to-12-week exercise training intervention found insulin resistance significantly improved even though BMI did not significantly reduce (Brown et al. 2009). It seems that even if weight loss is modest after exercise, the loss of visceral fat—which is more metabolically problematic than subcutaneous fat—is the key, as well as the building of muscle mass, which improves insulin resistance.

Inactive women with PCOS are more likely to have mild depression (Lamb et al. 2011). Exercising 3 days per week for six months improves body image in women with PCOS even if no weight is lost (Liao et al. 2008). Liao et al. found that brisk walking improved body image, despite no change in BMI. Saremi and Kazemi (2016) randomised 22 women with PCOS into either 10 weeks of aerobic exercise (~35 mins per week, 3 days per week) or a no-intervention control group, and found significant benefits for anxiety and depression ($p < 0.05$) with the intervention.

Based on review of 18 papers, Shetty et al. (2017) advise that health benefits in PCOS will be seen by following a programme of exercise based on 12–24 weeks of: aerobic training (e.g. bicycle) for ~40 minutes, 5 days per week, and weight training (e.g. dumbbells for biceps etc.) ~40 minutes, 2–3 days per week. These exercises should be done after a warm-up of at least 5–10 minutes, and afterwards, a cool-down period of calisthenics for 5–10 minutes. However this paper doesn't say how much weight might be lost.

Kirthika et al. (2019) cite an exercise specialist working in integrated medical care, who suggests that a minimum of 30 minutes of exercise (aerobic exercise and/or resistance training) 5 days per week should be sufficient for women suffering from PCOS to avoid the long-term complications of PCOS. However no research evidence was presented to support this suggestion.

A one-day education group for women with PCOS improved QoL, but not exercise behaviour, 12 months later (Mani et al. 2018). Compared to the 'usual care' group, participants randomised to the structured education programme had significantly improved QoL for emotions, QoL for fertility, QoL for weight, sense of control, mental well-being, and understanding of PCOS. These structured education events are probably especially useful to women without access to informed advice from the healthcare providers.

In a study of moderate to vigorous physical activity with 35 young women (aged 12–21) with PCOS, Michael et al. (2015) found that most participants exercised for around 10 minutes per day, and although parental assessments of depression were correlated with activity duration, the self-reported depression scores of the young women were not related to activity duration.

On a methodological point, most studies mix exercise with other interventions such as diet (Conte et al. 2015). This makes sense in clinical terms, but makes it impossible to see the individual contribution of each element of the intervention. It could be that there is a synergistic effect, where the combination of parts creates something greater than each element alone. In any case, research that can identify the individual elements, as well as synergistic combinations of elements, would be useful.

Improving QoL When Obesity Is the Main Problem

Overall, there is at least some evidence that HRQoL is improved by weight loss in both women with PCOS (Hahn et al. 2006) and in the general population (Kolotkin et al. 2001). A 5% decrease in body weight (which is ~3.5 kg, 7.5 lbs for the average UK woman of 147 lbs) improves glucose tolerance, which in turn, improves reproductive and diabetic issues (Sirmans and Pate 2014), androgen production, due to improved insulin resistance (Goodman et al. 2015), visceral fat mass (Despres et al. 2001), metabolic and menstrual functioning (Knowler et al. 2002; Moran et al. 2006). These changes may reduce inflammation, which could improve mood (Farrell and Antoni 2010).

Special Diets for PCOS

As mentioned in Chap. 5, reactive hypoglycaemia, typically mid-afternoon and after meals, may contribute to weight gain in PCOS (Magnotti and Futterweit 2007). This might happen because insulin induces the production of androgens, which in turn, increase visceral fat (Stanley and Misra 2008). A low glycemic index (GI) diet has been suggested as a way of controlling this problem. Galletly et al. (2007) and Herriot et al. (2008) found benefits of this diet for women with PCOS in relation to mood. Marsh et al. (2010) found that for moderately overweight women with PCOS, the low-GI diet significantly improved insulin resistance, menstruation (probably due to improved insulin sensitivity), and PCOSQ for emotions. The findings may have been stronger if there were not such a large dropout from this study, demonstrating again the importance of adherence in studies that make demands of participants' lifestyle.

Galletly et al. (2007) randomly allocated women with PCOS to either a low-carbohydrate high-protein diet for 16 weeks, or a high-carbohydrate low-protein diet. Despite there being no difference in the resulting weight loss, there were significant improvements in depression and self-esteem in the low-carbohydrate high-protein group. Farrell and Antoni (2010) suggest that this effect might be because women with PCOS are possibly more at risk of greater proinflammatory marker secretion after a high-carbohydrate meal than are healthy women.

Other Treatments for Weight Loss

Two relatively demanding diets used in non-PCOS populations have potential benefits for PCOS. One is the extreme calorie-controlled diet that Lim et al. (2011) found could, apparently, reverse type 2 diabetes. A similar diet has been piloted for obese women who want to lose weight in order to become pregnant (Brackenridge et al. 2018). Diets of this kind need to be undertaken with medical supervision.

A systematic review assessed which complementary medicine worked best for weight loss in the general population (Pittler and Ernst 2005).

The authors compared acupuncture, acupressure, dietary supplements, homeopathy, and hypnotherapy. They found that the two most effective methods were hypnotherapy and dietary supplements/stimulants. However, the supplements had the disadvantage of side effects, such as insomnia, anxiety, and palpitations.

Conclusion

The evidence presented in this chapter should be quite encouraging, in that the few studies that have been conducted appear to show that CBT, relaxation, diet, and exercise all find evidence of improving mental health aspects of PCOS. However more could be done to find out how to best tailor generic interventions to the specific and complex needs of women with PCOS. For example, we know from research in the general population that CBT and hypnotherapy combined can improve weight loss (Kirsch et al. 1995), and it would be interesting to see how well this works for women with PCOS.

A key time for weight loss interventions is not so much prior to trying to become pregnant, but prior to adolescence, when the child who is at risk of developing PCOS might be able to prevent this happening by taking a healthy interest in exercise and diet. It could be that a health promotion campaign, based on a model like the IMBP, aimed at parents with a familial history of PCOS and their children, has the potential to help children achieve a healthy weight before reaching puberty.

We have also seen that relaxation therapy can be delivered with some benefits to mental health relatively easily on a CD (Stefanaki et al. 2015). Ease of delivery is important when demanding interventions are associated with large dropout rates of 50%. Ensuring adherence, either by increasing the motivation of participants, identifying signs of potential dropout at initial recruitment (using the IMBP), or making the interventions as easy as possibly, could be useful in avoiding dropout. Individual therapy is more expensive than group therapy, and it would be useful to see how well each compares in terms of outcomes for women with PCOS. Sometimes groups can add a dynamic that helps with therapy and lowers dropout, though individual therapy is often thought to give better outcomes (Sin and Lyubomirsky 2009).

In the absence of expertise from individual health professionals, or being able to take part in longer-term interventions, structured education events (e.g. Mani et al. 2018) could be useful. These would be delivered by experts in PCOS, who could travel to hospitals and health centres, delivering their intervention to groups of women with PCOS.

Expert Opinions

Experts on psychological aspects of PCOS agree that mental health care should be an integral part of the healthcare provision for women with PCOS. In their review, Farrell and Antoni state that 'medical management of PCOS would greatly benefit from inclusion of psychological and behavioural approaches' (Farrell and Antoni 2010, p. 1565). In their review of the literature on psychological issues in PCOS, Himelein and Thatcher (2006) suggest that the initial evaluation of women with PCOS should include assessment of mental health, especially depression and abnormal eating patterns. The position statement by Dokras et al. (2018) further recommends that even if the initial test result indicates no mental health problems, repeat screening should be done for 'high-risk women such as those with anxiety, obesity, diabetes, and family history of depression and those in the postpartum period' (Dokras et al. 2018, p. 891). Appropriate referral should be made for those whose assessment suggests the need. One of the four recommendations in the guideline on the assessment and treatment of PCOS by Teede et al. (2018) is 'increasing focus on education, lifestyle modification, emotional wellbeing and quality'. But therein lies a critical issue for all concerned with PCOS; as stated by Teede et al.: 'there remains a large research gap. We agree that the current limited PCOS research funding is disproportionate to the significant social, health and economic burden of PCOS on the Australian population and health system' (Teede et al. 2019, p. 285). Given that the rates of moderate-to-severe anxiety in PCOS are 44.9%, and for depression are 25% (based on my calculations in Chaps. 2 and 3 of the data in Cooney et al. 2017), is important to focus screening and treatment on anxiety as well as depression. To do this probably requires greater understanding of the complex psychobiological interplay in PCOS, such as hypoglycaemia (Barry et al. 2011) and the role of adrenal androgens (Barry et al. 2017).

References

Abdollahi, L. (2016). *The effect of cognitive-behavioral therapy (CBT) on the quality of life and psychological fatigue in women with polycystic ovarian syndrome: A randomized control trial.* Doctoral dissertation, School of Nursing and Midwifery, Tabriz University of Medical Sciences.

Amianto, F., Ottone, L., Daga, G. A., & Fassino, S. (2015). Binge-eating disorder diagnosis and treatment: A recap in front of DSM-5. *BMC Psychiatry, 15*(1), 70.

Arasu, A., Moran, L. J., Robinson, T., Boyle, J., & Lim, S. (2019). Barriers and facilitators to weight and lifestyle management in women with polycystic ovary syndrome: General practitioners' perspectives. *Nutrients, 11*(5), 1024.

Barry, J. A., Hardiman, P. J., Saxby, B. K., & Kuczmierczyk, A. (2011). Testosterone and mood dysfunction in women with polycystic ovarian syndrome compared to subfertile controls. *Journal of Psychosomatic Obstetrics and Gynecology, 32*(2), 104–111.

Barry, J. A., Leite, N., Sivarajah, N., Keevil, B., Owen, L., Miranda, L. C., ... Hardiman, P. (2017). Relaxation and guided imagery significantly reduces androgen levels and distress in polycystic ovary syndrome: Pilot study. *Contemporary Hypnosis and Integrative Therapy, 32*(1), 21–29.

Benson, S., Arck, P. C., Tan, S., Hahn, S., Mann, K., Rifaie, N., ... Elsenbruch, S. (2009). Disturbed stress responses in women with polycystic ovary syndrome. *Psychoneuroendocrinology, 34*, 727–735.

Brackenridge, L., Finer, N., Batterham, R. L., Pedram, K., Ding, T., Stephenson, J., ... Hardiman, P. (2018). Pre-pregnancy weight loss in women with obesity requesting removal of their intra-uterine contraceptive device in order to conceive: A pilot study of full meal replacement. *Clinical Obesity, 8*(4), 244–249.

Brown, P. J. (1991). Culture and the evolution of obesity. *Human Nature, 2*, 31–57.

Brown, A. J., Setji, T. L., Sanders, L. L., Lowry, K. P., Otvos, J. D., Kraus, W. E., & Svetkey, P. L. (2009). Effects of exercise on lipoprotein particles in women with polycystic ovary syndrome. *Medicine and Science in Sports and Exercise, 41*, 497–504.

Cesta, C. E., Månsson, M., Palm, C., Lichtenstein, P., Iliadou, A. N., & Landén, M. (2016). Polycystic ovary syndrome and psychiatric disorders: Co-morbidity and heritability in a nationwide Swedish cohort. *Psychoneuroendocrinology, 73*, 196–203.

Cinar, N., Harmanci, A., Demir, B., & Yildiz, B. O. (2012). Effect of an oral contraceptive on emotional distress, anxiety and depression of women with polycystic ovary syndrome: A prospective study. *Human Reproduction, 27*, 1840–1845.

Clayton, W. J., Lipton, M., Elford, J., Rustin, M., & Sherr, L. (2005). A randomized controlled trial of laser treatment among hirsute women with polycystic ovary syndrome. *The British Journal of Dermatology, 152*, 986–992.

Conte, F., Banting, L., Teede, H. J., & Stepto, N. K. (2015). Mental health and physical activity in women with polycystic ovary syndrome: A brief review. *Sports Medicine, 45*(4), 497–504.

Cooney, L. G., & Dokras, A. (2017). Depression and anxiety in polycystic ovary syndrome: Etiology and treatment. *Current Psychiatry Reports, 19*(11), 83.

Cooney, L. G., Lee, I., Sammel, M. D., & Dokras, A. (2017). High prevalence of moderate and severe depressive and anxiety symptoms in polycystic ovary syndrome: A systematic review and meta-analysis. *Human Reproduction, 32*(5), 1075–1091.

Cooney, L. G., Milman, L. W., Hantsoo, L., Kornfield, S., Sammel, M. D., Allison, K. C., ... Dokras, A. (2018). Cognitive-behavioral therapy improves weight loss and quality of life in women with polycystic ovary syndrome: A pilot randomized clinical trial. *Fertility and Sterility, 110*(1), 161–171.

Correa, J. B., Sperry, S. L., & Darkes, J. (2015). A case report demonstrating the efficacy of a comprehensive cognitive-behavioral therapy approach for treating anxiety, depression, and problematic eating in polycystic ovarian syndrome. *Archives of Women's Mental Health, 18*(4), 649–654.

Cruess, D. G., Antoni, M. H., McGregor, B. A., Kilbourn, K. M., Boyers, A. E., Alferi, S. M., ... Kumar, M. (2000). Cognitive-behavioral stress management reduces serum cortisol by enhancing positive contributions among women being treated for early stage breast cancer. *Psychosomatic Medicine, 62*, 304–308.

Cruess, D., Antoni, M. H., Mahendra, K., McGregor, B., Alferi, S., Boyers, A., ... Kilbourn, K. (2001). Effects of stress management on testosterone levels in women with early-stage breast cancer. *International Journal of Behavioral Medicine, 8*, 194–207.

Cully, J. A., & Teten, A. L. (2008). *A therapist's guide to brief cognitive behavioral therapy*. Houston, TX: Department of Veterans Affairs South Central MIRECC.

Danese, A., & Tan, M. (2014). Childhood maltreatment and obesity: Systematic review and meta-analysis. *Molecular Psychiatry, 19*(5), 544.

David, D., Cotet, C., Matu, S., Mogoase, C., & Stefan, S. (2018). 50 years of rational-emotive and cognitive-behavioral therapy: A systematic review and meta-analysis. *Journal of Clinical Psychology, 74*(3), 304–318.

Deng, G., & Cassileth, B. R. (2005). Integrative oncology: Complementary therapies for pain, anxiety, and mood disturbance. *CA: A Cancer Journal for Clinicians, 55*(2), 109–116.

Despres, J. P., Lemieux, I., & Prud'homme, D. (2001). Treatment of obesity: Need to focus on high risk abdominally obese patients. *BMJ, 322*, 716–720.

DiClemente, C. C., & Prochaska, J. O. (1982). Self-change and therapy change of smoking behavior: A comparison of processes of change in cessation and maintenance. *Addictive Behaviors, 7*(2), 133–142.

Dokras, A., Sarwer, D. B., Allison, K. C., Milman, L., Kris-Etherton, P. M., Kunselman, A. R., … Fleming, J. (2016). Weight loss and lowering androgens predict improvements in health-related quality of life in women with PCOS. *The Journal of Clinical Endocrinology & Metabolism, 101*(8), 2966–2974.

Dokras, A., Stener-Victorin, E., Yildiz, B. O., Li, R., Ottey, S., Shah, D., … & Teede, H. (2018). Androgen Excess-Polycystic Ovary Syndrome Society: position statement on depression, anxiety, quality of life, and eating disorders in polycystic ovary syndrome. *Fertility and Sterility, 109*(5), 888–899.

Dunaif, A., & Fauser, B. C. (2013). Renaming PCOS—A two-state solution. *The Journal of Clinical Endocrinology & Metabolism, 98*(11), 4325–4328.

Elizabeth, M., Leslie, N. S., & Critch, E. A. (2009). Managing polycystic ovary syndrome: A cognitive behavioral strategy. *Nursing for Women's Health, 13*(4), 292–300.

Ezeh, U., Yildiz, B. O., & Azziz, R. (2013). Referral bias in defining the phenotype and prevalence of obesity in polycystic ovary syndrome. *The Journal of Clinical Endocrinology and Metabolism, 98*(6), E1088–E1096.

Farrell, K., & Antoni, M. H. (2010). Insulin resistance, obesity, inflammation, and depression in polycystic ovary syndrome: Biobehavioral mechanisms and interventions. *Fertility and Sterility, 94*(5), 1565–1574.

Fernandez, R. C., Moore, V. M., Van Ryswyk, E. M., Varcoe, T. J., Rodgers, R. J., March, W. A., … Davies, M. J. (2018). Sleep disturbances in women with polycystic ovary syndrome: Prevalence, pathophysiology, impact and management strategies. *Nature and Science of Sleep, 10*, 45.

Fishbein, M., Triandis, H. C., Kanfer, F. H., Becker, M., Middlestadt, S. E., & Eichler, A. (2001). Factors influencing behavior and behavior change. *Handbook of Health Psychology*, 3–17.

Fruzzetti, F., Perini, D., Russo, M., Bucci, F., & Gadducci, A. (2017). Comparison of two insulin sensitizers, metformin and myo-inositol, in women with polycystic ovary syndrome (PCOS). *Gynecological Endocrinology, 33*(1), 39–42.

Galletly, C., Moran, L., Noakes, M., Clifton, P., Tomlinson, L., & Norman, R. (2007). Psychological benefits of a high-protein, low-carbohydrate diet in obese women with polycystic ovary syndrome—A pilot study. *Appetite, 49*(3), 590–593.

Gallinelli, A., Matteo, M. L., Volpe, A., & Facchinetti, F. (2000). Autonomic and neuroendocrine responses to stress in patients with functional hypothalamic secondary amenorrhea. *Fertility and Sterility, 73*, 812–816.

Gibson-Helm, M., Teede, H., Dunaif, A., & Dokras, A. (2017). Delayed diagnosis and a lack of information associated with dissatisfaction in women with polycystic ovary syndrome. *The Journal of Clinical Endocrinology & Metabolism, 102*(2), 604–612.

Godfrey, K. M., Gallo, L. C., & Afari, N. (2015). Mindfulness-based interventions for binge eating: A systematic review and meta-analysis. *Journal of Behavioral Medicine, 38*(2), 348–362.

Graff, S. K., Mario, F. M., Ziegelmann, P., & Spritzer, P. M. (2016). Effects of orlistat vs. metformin on weight loss-related clinical variables in women with PCOS: Systematic review and meta-analysis. *International Journal of Clinical Practice, 70*(6), 450–461.

Hahn, S., Janssen, O. E., Tan, S., Pleger, K., Mann, K., Schedlowski, M., … Elsenbruch, S. (2005). Clinical and psychological correlates of quality-of-life in polycystic ovary syndrome. *European Journal of Endocrinology, 153*, 853–860.

Hahn, S., Benson, S., Elsenbruch, S., Pleger, K., Tan, S., Mann, K., … Janssen, O. E. (2006). Metformin treatment of polycystic ovary syndrome improves health-related quality-of-life, emotional distress and sexuality. *Human Reproduction, 21*, 1925–1934.

Harrison, C. L., Lombard, C. B., Moran, L. J., & Teede, H. J. (2010). Exercise therapy in polycystic ovary syndrome: A systematic review. *Human Reproduction Update, 17*(2), 171–183.

Herriot, A. M., Whitcroft, S., & Jeanes, Y. (2008). An retrospective audit of patients with polycystic ovary syndrome: The effects of a reduced glycaemic load diet. *Journal of Human Nutrition and Dietetics, 21*(4), 337–345.

Himelein, M. J., & Thatcher, S. S. (2006). Polycystic ovary syndrome and mental health: A review. *Obstetrical & Gynecological Survey, 61*, 723–732.

Hopkins, C. S., Kimble, L. P., Hodges, H. F., Koci, A. F., & Mills, B. B. (2019). A mixed-methods study of coping and depression in adolescent girls with polycystic ovary syndrome. *Journal of the American Association of Nurse Practitioners, 31*(3), 189–197.

Huber-Buchholz, M. M., Carey, D. G. P., & Norman, R. J. (1999). Restoration of reproductive potential by lifestyle modification in obese polycystic ovary syndrome: Role of insulin sensitivity and luteinizing hormone. *The Journal of Clinical Endocrinology & Metabolism, 84*(4), 1470–1474.

Jakubowski, K. P., Black, J. J., El Nokali, N. E., Belendiuk, K. A., Hannon, T. S., Arslanian, S. A., & Rofey, D. L. (2012). Parents' readiness to change affects BMI reduction outcomes in adolescents with polycystic ovary syndrome. *Journal of Obesity, 2012*, 298067.

Jones, G. L., Hall, J. M., Balen, A. H., & Ledger, W. L. (2008). Health-related quality of life measurement in women with polycystic ovary syndrome: A systematic review. *Human Reproduction Update, 14*, 15–25.

Kaltsas, G. A., Isidori, A. M., Kola, B. P., Skelly, R. H., Chew, S. L., Jenkins, P. J., ... Besser, G. M. (2003). The value of the low-dose dexamethasone suppression test in the differential diagnosis of hyperandrogenism in women. *The Journal of Clinical Endocrinology & Metabolism, 88*(6), 2634–2643.

Keski-Rahkonen, A., Bulik, C. M., Pietiläinen, K. H., Rose, R. J., Kaprio, J., & Rissanen, A. (2007). Eating styles, overweight and obesity in young adult twins. *European Journal of Clinical Nutrition, 61*, 822–829.

Kirsch, I., Montgomery, G., & Sapirstein, G. (1995). Hypnosis as an adjunct to cognitive-behavioral psychotherapy: A meta-analysis. *Journal of Consulting and Clinical Psychology, 63*(2), 214.

Kirthika, S. V., Paul, J., Sudhakar, S., & Selvam, P. S. (2019). Polycystic ovarian syndrome-interventions for the emerging public health challenge: A scoping review. *Drug Invention Today, 12*(3), 1–4.

Knowler, W. C., Barrett-Connor, E., Fowler, S. E., Hamman, R. F., Lachin, J. M., Walker, E. A., ... Diabetes Prevention Program Research Group. (2002). Reduction in the incidence of type 2 diabetes with lifestyle intervention or metformin. *The New England Journal of Medicine, 346*, 393–403.

Kolotkin, R. L., Meter, K., & Williams, G. R. (2001). Quality of life and obesity. *Obesity Reviews, 2*, 219–229.

Lamb, J. D., Johnstone, E. B., Rousseau, J. A., Jones, C. L., Pasch, L. A., Cedars, M. I., & Huddleston, H. G. (2011). Physical activity in women with polycystic ovary syndrome: Prevalence, predictors, and positive health associations. *American Journal of Obstetrics and Gynecology, 204*(4), 352–3e1.

Liao, L. M., Nesic, J., Chadwick, P. M., Brooke-Wavell, K., & Prelevic, G. M. (2008). Exercise and body image distress in overweight and obese women with polycystic ovary syndrome: A pilot investigation. *Gynecological Endocrinology, 24,* 555–561.

Lim, E. L., Hollingsworth, K. G., Aribisala, B. S., Chen, M. J., Mathers, J. C., & Taylor, R. (2011). Reversal of type 2 diabetes: Normalisation of beta cell function in association with decreased pancreas and liver triacylglycerol. *Diabetologia, 54*(10), 2506–2514.

Magnotti, M., & Futterweit, W. (2007). Obesity and the polycystic ovary syndrome. *Medical Clinics of North America, 91*(6), 1151–1168.

Mani, H., Chudasama, Y., Hadjiconstantinou, M., Bodicoat, D. H., Edwardson, C., Levy, M. J., ... Khunti, K. (2018). Structured education programme for women with polycystic ovary syndrome: A randomised controlled trial. *Endocrine Connections, 7*(1), 26–35.

Månsson, M., Holte, J., Landin-Wilhelmsen, K., Dahlgren, E., Johansson, A., & Landén, M. (2008). Women with polycystic ovary syndrome are often depressed or anxious—A case control study. *Psychoneuroendocrinology, 33*(8), 1132–1138.

Marsh, K. A., Steinbeck, K. S., Atkinson, F. S., Petocz, P., & Brand-Miller, J. C. (2010). Effect of a low glycemic index compared with a conventional healthy diet on polycystic ovary syndrome. *The American Journal of Clinical Nutrition, 92*(1), 83–92.

McCook, J. G., Reame, N. E., & Thatcher, S. S. (2005). Health-related quality of life issues in women with polycystic ovary syndrome. *Journal of Obstetric, Gynecologic, and Neonatal Nursing, 34,* 12–20.

Michael, J. C., El Nokali, N. E., Black, J. J., & Rofey, D. L. (2015). Mood and ambulatory monitoring of physical activity patterns in youth with polycystic ovary syndrome. *Journal of Pediatric and Adolescent Gynecology, 28*(5), 369–372.

Moeller, L. V., Lindhardt, C. L., Andersen, M. S., Glintborg, D., & Ravn, P. (2019). Motivational interviewing in obese women with polycystic ovary syndrome—A pilot study. *Gynecological Endocrinology, 35*(1), 76–80.

Moran, L. J., Noakes, M., Clifton, P. M., Tomlinson, L., Galletly, C., & Norman, R. J. (2003). Dietary composition in restoring reproductive and metabolic physiology in overweight women with polycystic ovary syndrome. *The Journal of Clinical Endocrinology and Metabolism, 88,* 812–819.

Moran, L. J., Brinkworth, G., Noakes, M., & Norman, R. J. (2006). Effects of lifestyle modification in polycystic ovary syndrome. *Reproductive Biomedicine Online, 12*, 569–578.

Naqvi, S. H., Moore, A., Bevilacqua, K., Lathief, S., Williams, J., Naqvi, N., & Pal, L. (2015). Predictors of depression in women with polycystic ovary syndrome. *Archives of Women's Mental Health, 18*(1), 95–101.

NHS. (2016). *Clinical depression: Treatment.* Retrieved May 29, 2019, from https://www.nhs.uk/conditions/clinical-depression/treatment/.

NHS. (2019). *Cognitive behavioural therapy (CBT).* Retrieved May 19, 2019, from https://www.nhs.uk/conditions/cognitive-behavioural-therapy-cbt/.

NICE. (2018). *Depression in adults: Treatment and management.* Retrieved May 29, 2019, from https://www.nice.org.uk/guidance/gid-cgwave0725/documents/full-guideline-updated.

Noll, J. G., Zeller, M. H., Trickett, P. K., & Putnam, F. W. (2007). Obesity risk for female victims of childhood sexual abuse: A prospective study. *Pediatrics, 120*(1), e61–e67.

Palomba, S., Giallauria, F., Falbo, A., Russo, T., Oppedisano, R., Tolino, A., … Orio, F. (2008). Structured exercise training programme versus hypocaloric hyperproteic diet in obese polycystic ovary syndrome patients with anovulatory infertility: A 24-week pilot study. *Human Reproduction, 23*, 642–650.

Pittler, M. H., & Ernst, E. (2005). Complementary therapies for reducing body weight: A systematic review. *International Journal of Obesity, 29*(9), 1030.

Rasgon, N. L., Rao, R. C., Hwang, S., Altshuler, L. L., Elman, S., Zuckerbrow-Miller, J., & Korenman, S. G. (2003). Depression in women with polycystic ovary syndrome: Clinical and biochemical correlates. *Journal of Affective Disorders, 74*, 299–304.

Rofey, D. L., Szigethy, E. M., Noll, R. B., Dahl, R. E., Lobst, E., & Arslanian, S. A. (2008). Cognitive–behavioral therapy for physical and emotional disturbances in adolescents with polycystic ovary syndrome: A pilot study. *Journal of Pediatric Psychology, 34*(2), 156–163.

Rofey, D. L., Szigethy, E. M., Noll, R. B., Dahl, R. E., Lobst, E., & Arslanian, S. A. (2009). Cognitive-behavioral therapy for physical and emotional disturbances in adolescents with polycystic ovary syndrome: A pilot study. *Journal of Pediatric Psychology, 34*, 156–163.

Rofey, D. L., El Nokali, N. E., Foster, L. J. J., Seiler, E., McCauley, H. L., & Miller, E. (2018). Weight loss trajectories and adverse childhood experience among obese adolescents with polycystic ovary syndrome. *Journal of Pediatric and Adolescent Gynecology, 31*(4), 372–375.

Sam, S. (2007). Obesity and polycystic ovary syndrome. *Obesity Management, 3*, 69–73.

Saremi, A., & Kazemi, M. (2016). The effect of an aerobic training period on mental health and depression in Iranian women with polycystic ovary syndrome. *Complementary Medicine Journal of Faculty of Nursing & Midwifery, 6*(18), 1420–1431.

Shetty, D., Chandrasekaran, B., Singh, A. W., & Oliverraj, J. (2017). Exercise in polycystic ovarian syndrome: An evidence-based review. *Saudi Journal of Sports Medicine, 17*(3), 123.

Sin, N. L., & Lyubomirsky, S. (2009). Enhancing well-being and alleviating depressive symptoms with positive psychology interventions: A practice-friendly meta-analysis. *Journal of Clinical Psychology, 65*(5), 467–487.

Sirmans, S. M., & Pate, K. A. (2014). Epidemiology, diagnosis, and management of polycystic ovary syndrome. *Clinical Epidemiology, 6*, 1.

Spielberger, C. D., Sydeman, S. J., Owen, A. E., & Marsh, B. J. (1999). Measuring anxiety and anger with the State-Trait Anxiety Inventory (STAI) and the State-Trait Anger Expression Inventory (STAXI). In M. E. Maruish (Ed.), *The use of psychological testing for treatment planning and outcomes assessment* (pp. 993–1021). Mahwah, NJ: Lawrence Erlbaum Associates Publishers.

Stanley, T., & Misra, M. (2008). Polycystic ovary syndrome in obese adolescents. *Current Opinion in Endocrinology, Diabetes, and Obesity, 15*, 30–36.

Stapinska-Syniec, A., Grabowska, K., Szpotanska-Sikorska, M., & Pietrzak, B. (2018). Depression, sexual satisfaction, and other psychological issues in women with polycystic ovary syndrome. *Gynecological Endocrinology, 34*(7), 597–600.

Stefanaki, C., Bacopoulou, F., Livadas, S., Kandaraki, A., Karachalios, A., Chrousos, G. P., & Diamanti-Kandarakis, E. (2015). Impact of a mindfulness stress management program on stress, anxiety, depression and quality of life in women with polycystic ovary syndrome: A randomized controlled trial. *Stress, 18*(1), 57–66.

Stunkard, A. J., Faith, A. S., & Allison, K. C. (2003). Depression and obesity. *Biological Psychiatry, 54*, 330–337.

Sullivan, M. (2017, August 31). What's in a name? *Clinical Endocrinology News.*

Teede, H. J., Misso, M. L., Costello, M. F., Dokras, A., Laven, J., Moran, L., … Norman, R. J. (2018). Recommendations from the international evidence-based guideline for the assessment and management of polycystic ovary syndrome. *Human Reproduction, 33*(9), 1602–1618.

Teede, H. J., Norman, R. J., & Garad, R. M. (2019). A new evidence-based guideline for assessment and management of polycystic ovary syndrome. *The Medical Journal of Australia, 210*(6), 285.

Thessaloniki ESHRE/ASRM-Sponsored PCOS Consensus Workshop Group. (2008). Consensus on infertility treatment related to polycystic ovary syndrome. *Human Reproduction, 23*, 462–477.

Thompson, J. K., Heinberg, L. J., Altabe, M., & Tantleff-Dunn, S. (1999). *Exacting beauty: Theory, assessment, and treatment of body image disturbance.* Washington, DC: American Psychological Association.

Thomson, R. L., Buckley, J. D., Lim, S. S., Noakes, M., Clifton, P. M., Norman, R. J., & Brinkworth, G. D. (2010). Lifestyle management improves quality of life and depression in overweight and obese women with polycystic ovary syndrome. *Fertility and sterility, 94*(5), 1812–1816.

Trent, M., Austin, S. B., Rich, M., & Gordon, C. M. (2005). Overweight status of adolescent girls with polycystic ovary syndrome: Body mass index as mediator of quality of life. *Ambulatory Pediatrics, 5*, 107–111.

Vgontzas, A. N. (2008). Does obesity play a major role in the pathogenesis of sleep apnoea and its associated manifestations via inflammation, visceral adiposity, and insulin resistance? *Archives of Physiology and Biochemistry, 114*, 211–223.

Wake, D. J., Strand, M., Rask, E., Westerbacka, J., Livingstone, D. E., Soderberg, S., … Walker, B. R. (2007). Intra-adipose sex steroid metabolism and body fat distribution in idiopathic human obesity. *Clinical Endocrinology, 66*, 440–446.

Wang, K. C., & Zane, L. T. (2008). Recent advances in acne vulgaris research: Insights and clinical implications. *Advances in Dermatology, 24*, 197–209.

9

Conclusion

Abstract Perhaps by now, having read the previous chapters, you will understand why PCOS is such a fascinating topic, and—like me—you might be perplexed as to why it is so neglected, especially given the scale and impact of this syndrome. In this concluding section, I hazard a guess as to why this situation exists how the situation might be remedied, and what they key points are for the future of PCOS research and practice.

Keywords Research community • Psychologist • Policy • Public health

Psychologists Say It's Good to Talk, So Why Aren't Psychologists Talking About PCOS?

In the preface I highlighted how little interest amongst psychologists there is in PCOS. This is extraordinary, especially when most psychologists are women, and probably 10% or more themselves have PCOS. So why the lack of interest? One possibility is that PCOS is an embarrassing condition and women simply don't want to talk about it. This is an interesting idea, because it is commonly thought that when women feel

© The Author(s) 2019   225
J. A. Barry, *Psychological Aspects of Polycystic Ovary Syndrome,*
https://doi.org/10.1007/978-3-030-30290-0_9

distressed they want to talk about it. Indeed research evidence supports this view (e.g. Holloway et al. 2018). However, perhaps there are exceptions to this rule. For example, it is surprisingly uncommon knowledge that a woman's fertility—even a very healthy woman—drops steeply after the age of 35. Indeed women's fertility was infamously described in the media as 'falling off a cliff' after age 35 (Tran 2014). Not only are women not generally aware of this fact, but many seem actively hostile to talking about it. Similarly, miscarriage rates are around 1 in 4 even in healthy pregnancies, but women don't tend to know about this. Perhaps it is just too painful to discuss? These are just two examples of potentially many where women are reluctant to discuss their feelings about issues. The common factor is that they relate to their fertility and reproduction—a very central part of their sense of being a woman. It could be that female psychologists are not immune to this phenomenon.

It's true that in general when men face emotional problems especially ones that impact their identity as men, such as unemployment—they tend not to want to talk about it, and prefer to try to fix the problem themselves (Holloway et al. 2018). However it is true that men benefit from having their troubles listened to, which is probably why they are often urged in public campaigns to 'just open up'. This very direct approach, of simply urging men to do what many of them they clearly don't want to, is probably not the best thought-through strategy. Liddon et al. (2019) suggest various indirect approaches to helping men get to the point where they want to discuss their feelings, and perhaps some creative thinking is needed in order to get women to want to talk about their PCOS. It could be that, for example, a solution-focused approach could be utilised rather than an emotion-focused approach, for example taking a step-by-step approach to fixing the medical problems of PCOS as a way of fixing the emotional aspects. This solution-focused approach is generally a more male-typical approach to dealing with problems, but can work for women too. Indeed this might be what is being demonstrated in the US by the very successful campaigning of the *PCOS Challenge* charity, which takes proactive steps to highlight the issues faced by women with PCOS, and encourages the US government and health institutes to take positive action to remedy the problem of PCOS.

Chapter 1 gave some idea of the difficulty of working on a medical condition that is so complex that it's even difficult to find a suitable name for it. Finding more suitable names derived more directly from the individual phenotypes could be considered (Dunaif and Fauser 2013). Renaming might reduce fear and misunderstanding too (e.g. should they be called 'cysts'?). Renaming might reduce stigma, for example, the term 'neuroticism' has pejorative connotations, and might be changed to something that reflects its origins in lability of the HPA axis.

Breaking down the problem might help, including properly defining the various phenotypes, what causes them, and how we can treat them. This is a massive task and at present there is not only not the will, there is not even the awareness needed, to start this process.

What Are the Key Issues Facing PCOS Today?

One of the salient messages of Chap. 2 is that we need more clarity in how we define and discuss the causes and severity of depression in PCOS. A consensus on best practice around methodology would be useful.

Although the causes of depression in PCOS are possibly relatively straightforward (i.e. feeling low because of PCOS symptoms and issues such as obesity), Chap. 3 suggests that the role of anxiety in PCOS is more complex. Indeed it appears that the rates of moderate-to-severe anxiety in PCOS (44.9%) are higher than those of moderate-to-severe depression (25.0%), yet depression is more likely to be assessed than anxiety in PCOS research. Anxiety, and the related construct of 'neuroticism', are probably the tip of the iceberg for mood and metabolism in PCOS.

Chapter 4 demonstrates that there is a whole other body of literature on the psychological aspects of testosterone that have not been tapped into in our efforts to understand PCOS. Although the impact of elevated testosterone on health in women is generally negative, perhaps we should consider more the potential positive aspects of testosterone (e.g. mental rotation ability), not least because it might give hope to women who have this otherwise unrewarding condition.

Chapter 5, like Chap. 3, shows how the impact of insulin on mood via hypoglycaemia is one that could be relatively easily researched, and could have far-reaching benefits to physical and mental health.

For many women with PCOS, Chap. 6 cuts right to the heart of the problem of having PCOS. Improvements to fertility outcomes could have far-reaching benefits for these women, and with what we know now about AMH, and potential benefits of cetrorelix acetate, it could be that we might even be able to reduce the incidence of PCOS in the coming years.

Chapter 7 offers a large number of testable hypotheses for researchers in this complex field. For those willing and able (and funded) to take on such projects, much might be learned from exploring how well Figs. 7.1, 7.2, 7.3, and 7.4 map onto reality. Inevitably, the reality will be more complex than the map, but the research programmes may offer tangible benefits to scientists, healthcare practitioners, and women with PCOS.

It is perplexing that so few psychologists have taken any notice of PCOS. Chapter 8, shows that to date there are only four studies of CBT for PCOS, and one of these is a case study. This is a remarkable oversight by the psychology community. We can do better than this, and if we can begin to apply the knowledge and skills of psychologists to the massive problem of PCOS, the gains might be tremendous for women with PCOS, their families, and future generations who might not have to suffer in the same way from this condition.

References

Dunaif, A., & Fauser, B. C. (2013). Renaming PCOS—A two-state solution. *The Journal of Clinical Endocrinology & Metabolism, 98*(11), 4325–4328.

Holloway, K., Seager, M., & Barry, J. A. (2018). Are clinical psychologists, psychotherapists and counsellors overlooking the needs of their male clients. *Clinical Psychology Forum, 307*, 15–21.

Liddon, L., Kingerlee, R., Seager, M., & Barry, J. A. (2019). What are the factors that make a male-friendly therapy? In J. A. Barry, R. Kingerlee, M. J. Seager, & L. Sullivan (Eds.), *The Palgrave Handbook of Male Psychology and Mental Health*. London: Palgrave Macmillan.

Tran, M. (2014, June 2). Kirstie Allsopp tells young women: Ditch university and have a baby by 27. In *The Guardian* newspaper. Retrieved May 27, 2019, from https://www.theguardian.com/tv-and-radio/2014/jun/02/kirstie-allsop-young-women-ditch-university-baby-by-27.

Index

© The Author(s) 2019
J. A. Barry, *Psychological Aspects of Polycystic Ovary Syndrome*,
https://doi.org/10.1007/978-3-030-30290-0